Living & Well With Lung Cancer

Barbara Gitlitz, MD
Daniel Oh, MD
Amol Rao, MD
Stephen V. Liu, MD
O. Kenneth Macdonald, MD
Wayne T. Lamoreaux, MD
Robert K. Fairbanks, MD
Jason A. Call, MD
Heather Gabbert, MS, RD, LD, CD
Tess Taft, MSW, LICSW
Kathy Beach, RN
Christopher M. Lee, MD

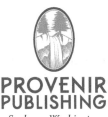

PROVENIR PUBLISHING

Spokane, Washington

The development of this patient handbook was
sponsored in part by an educational grant from:

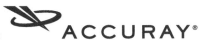
ACCURAY®

Living & Thriving With Lung Cancer

Published by Provenir Publishing, LLC, P. O. Box 211, Greenacres, WA 99016-0211

Production Credits

Lead Editor: Christopher Lee

Production Director: Amy Harman

Art Director and Illustration: Micah Harman

Cover Design: Micah Harman

Printing History: April 2013, First Edition.

www.provenirpublishing.com

This book is dedicated to our patients and their families,
who inspire us every day in their fight against cancer.

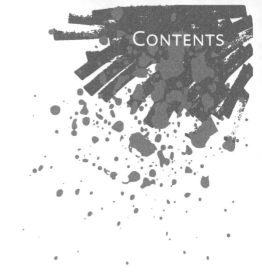

CONTENTS

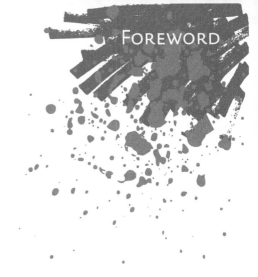

If you are holding this book in your hand, it is likely that you, a close family member, or close friend has been diagnosed with lung cancer. In most cases, this diagnosis is a shock and came from "out of the blue." You probably have 1000 questions floating around in your head; like how this illness will be treated, how you will feel, how this will affect your family and your work, and what should you do next. Any cancer diagnosis has an impact on many aspects of life. This is a fact for everyone. The goal of this book is to provide you with knowledge about your diagnosis and to assist in clarifying procedures, alleviate fears, and optimize your treatment. Our hope is that this is written in such a way that it is easy to understand and answers questions that commonly come up with a lung cancer diagnosis. We also have included a section on practical nutritional techniques that can add to your ability to heal, improve your immune system, and optimize your energy and overall health.

Cancers of the lung can affect patients in a wide variety of ways and require a team of physicians and health care providers to assist on this path of treatment.

The goal of this book is to compile experience and expertise in a way that can be easily interpreted. It is designed to provide rapid assistance in answering questions and to guide to you in your cancer journey.

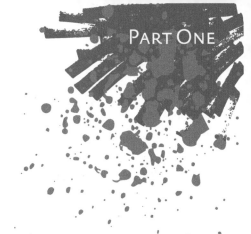
What Is Lung Cancer?

Cancer cells always start from a normal cell in the body that develops a series of genetic (DNA) mutations (changes). Lung cancer occurs when cells of the lung are damaged or mutated in a way which causes them to grow uncontrollably and unchecked. As these cells multiply, they form larger tumors and can spread by the blood or the lymphatic system to parts of the body outside of the lung.

fig. 1.1

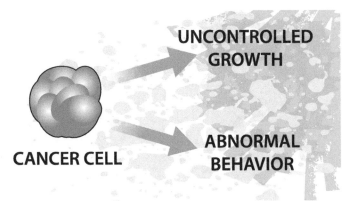

UNCONTROLLED GROWTH

CANCER CELL

ABNORMAL BEHAVIOR

Cancer cells start with abnormal DNA.

There are two main categories of lung cancer: **Non Small Cell Lung Cancer** and **Small Cell Lung Cancer**. A **Pathologist** (a doctor who specializes in distinguishing between tissue types) makes this distinction by **histology** (the way cells appear under a microscope). It is important to distinguish between these categories because the treatments and prognosis are very different.

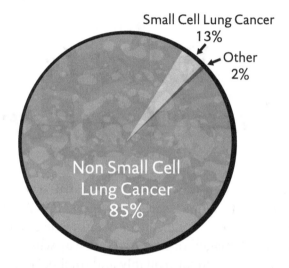

Small Cell Lung Cancer
13%

Other
2%

Non Small Cell
Lung Cancer
85%

fig. 1.2

Non Small Cell Lung Cancers account for about 85% of all lung cancers diagnosed. It is further subdivided by histology into 3 distinct subtypes:

1. *Adenocarcinoma*: Usually occurs on the outer areas of the lung, resembles the mucus producing cells of the lung.

2. *Squamous Cell Carcinoma*: Usually occurs in the central areas of the lung, looks like the cells that line the air passages of the lung.

3. *Large Cell Carcinoma*: Usually occurs in the outer areas of the lung, appears larger than normal lung cells because of more fluid inside the cells.

Small Cell Lung Cancer accounts for about 13% of all lung cancers diagnosed and is a more aggressive type of lung cancer. They tend to grow quickly and spread to other organs at a more rapid pace. These cells appear small and blue under the microscope.

Lung cancers usually spread (metastasize) to adjacent lymph nodes first. The lymphatic vessels and lymph nodes are part of the immune system and help filter and drain excess fluid from all parts of the body. It is important to note that cancers that start in other organs and spread to the lung are *not* called lung cancer. They are called **metastases** from the cancer in which they started. For example, colon cancer that spreads to the lung is considered "metastatic colon cancer". The reverse is also true. Lung cancer that spreads to other organs (liver, adrenal glands, brain, or bone) is considered "metastatic lung cancer" even though it is now growing in another organ.

NURSE'S NOTE:

When a cancer metastasizes to another organ, this is usually a result of cancer cells entering the blood stream, traveling to another site in the body, and then forming new colonies by growing in other organs.

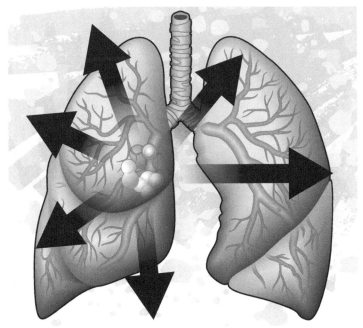

fig. 1.3

Lung cancer can metastasize (spread).

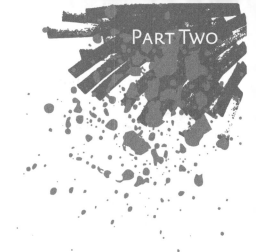

PART TWO

How Do I Know If I Have Lung Cancer And How Extensive Is It?

What are the common symptoms of lung cancer?

There are a variety of symptoms that may be caused by lung cancer. Although most of these are not specific to lung cancer, a combination of these symptoms and a thorough history of your risk factors may cause a doctor to suspect lung cancer. These symptoms of lung cancer can occur because of the effects from the tumor pushing and growing on the lung itself, effects on other areas of the body to where the lung cancer has spread, or because the tumor disrupts the normal function of the body or invades nerves which causes pain.

The following are common symptoms with diagnosis:

- Cough
- Coughing up of blood (hemoptysis)
- Shortness of breath
- Hoarseness / raspy voice
- Recurring lung infections
- Pain when taking deep breaths / rib pain
- Swelling of the neck / face / arms
- Bone pain
- Headaches / blurry vision / weakness
- Unexplained / unintentional weight loss
- Unexplained fevers
- Blood clots

What are the common causes of lung cancer?

When normal cells in the body are damaged, they usually die through a normal process. Cancer is caused when cell DNA is damaged or mutated in such a way that the cells divide uncontrollably and do not die. This DNA damage can occur due to a variety of environmental and genetic factors.

Smoking (cigarettes or a pipe) is a major contributor to the vast majority of lung cancer cases. The risk of cancer rises with the number of cigarettes and the number of years that someone has smoked. Second hand smoke may also increase the risk of developing lung cancer. However, lung cancer can also occur in people that have never smoked.

Other environmental risk factors include exposure to air pollution, coal, radon gas, asbestos, and radiation.

Some patients may also have a genetic predisposition to developing lung cancer due to the inheritance of genetic mutations from their family, but this is very rare.

What are the standard tests for diagnosis?

Imaging

The imaging work-up for lung cancer usually begins with an X-ray of the chest.

Depending on the findings, more detailed tests are usually performed, such as:

- *Computed Tomography (CT) Scan (also called a CAT scan)*: This is a machine that uses x-ray images from many different angles to generate a very detailed anatomic picture of the body and area of interest. Often, a dye called contrast is injected into the veins prior to the scan to improve the clarity of the images.

- *Positron Emission Tomography (PET) Scan*: This machine uses a type of radioactive material injected into the veins to show areas of high activity in the body. Because cancer cells are very active and divide quickly, they will often absorb more of the radioactive material and thus appear brighter on the images. The whole body can be imaged. It is often combined with a CT (CT/PET) scan to get even more precise information.

- *Bone Scan*: This scan uses radioactive material injected into the veins to show areas of bone damage that may occur from the spread of lung cancer.

fig. 2.1

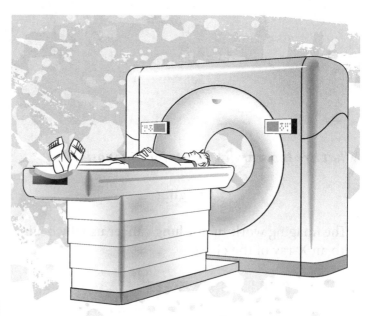

CT scans allow your doctors to map out the extent of the cancer spread.

Biopsy

After imaging studies have been performed, a biopsy (piece of tissue) of one of the sites of disease is required for diagnosis. This can be accomplished in several ways:

- *Bronchoscopic Biopsy*: If the tumor is inside or near some of the larger air passages of the lung, a pulmonologist (lung doctor) may be able to pass a scope (long, thin camera) through the mouth and into the airways to sample the necessary tissue using a small needle.

- *Image Guided Biopsy*: A Radiologist (doctor specializing in imaging scans) can use imaging like a CT scan or ultrasound to guide a needle to the site of the tumor to acquire a piece of tissue or a collection of fluid with a small needle.

fig. 2.2

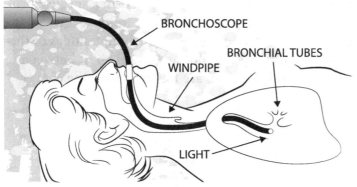

Bronchoscopy

This biopsy specimen will then be examined by a Pathologist to determine what cell type and what subset of cancer is present. Often, various characteristics of the cancer cells are examined in order to determine the best therapeutic options available.

How is Lung Cancer graded and staged?

Tumor grade is determined by how abnormal the cancer cells appear under the microscope. There are four severities of tumor Grade (numbered 1 through 4). The higher the tumor Grade the more aggressive the cancer is expected to be. Grade 1 tumors appear very much like normal cells whereas Grade 3–4 tumors appear very abnormal.

Stage is determined by the size of the primary lung tumor, the number and location of lymph nodes involved with lung cancer, and the areas of involvement if the cancer has spread to other organs. It is important to note that the stage and grade of a tumor are separate and different. Staging is important in guiding what the best treatment options are and also to determine prognosis. Staging is performed using the imaging studies mentioned in the previous section. A

NURSE'S NOTE:

It is important to let your doctor know if you are on blood thinners (including aspirin, Advil, and Aleve) prior to having a CT-guided biopsy. Blood thinners should be stopped prior to a biopsy.

NURSE'S NOTE:

A mediastinoscopy is done by a surgeon making a small incision in the chest and using a scope to look inside your chest and take samples of tissue. You will be asleep for this procedure.

thoracic surgeon may need to perform a surgical procedure called a **mediastinoscopy** to make an accurate determination about whether the lymph nodes of the mediastinum (the area in the central chest between the right and left lung) are involved with the cancer.

fig. 2.3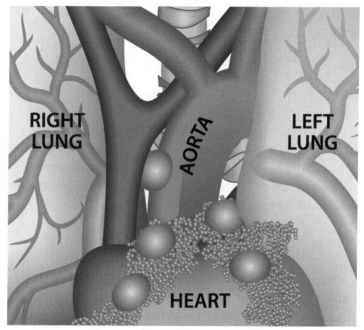

The Mediastinum is the anatomic area that contains lymph nodes between the lungs and above and behind the heart.

NON SMALL CELL LUNG CANCER STAGING

The simplified staging for non-small cell lung cancer is shown below, although a tumor stage may increase if it involves important lung structures such as major airways or the lining of the lung:

Stage I: The tumor is less than 5 cm in size, there are no lymph nodes involved, and there is no cancer in any other part of the body.

Stage IIA: The tumor is up to 5 cm in size and there are nearby lung lymph nodes involved with cancer, but there is no cancer in any other part of the body

OR: The tumor is between 5 and 7 cm in size; there is no lymph node involvement; and there is no cancer in any other part of the body.

Stage IIB: The tumor is between 5 and 7 cm, and there are nearby lung lymph nodes involved with the cancer. However, there is no cancer in any other part of the body

OR: The tumor is larger than 7 cm; there is no lymph node involvement; and there is no cancer in any other part of the body.

Stage IIIA: The tumor can be of any size, but the cancer has spread to lymph nodes around the major central airways or in the mediastinum on the same side of the lung as the primary tumor, and the cancer has not spread to other parts of the body

OR: The tumor has grown into the mediastinum or other vital structures

OR: There are several tumors in different lobes of the same lung.

Stage IIIB: The tumor can be of any size, but it has spread to lymph nodes on the opposite side of the primary lung tumor. However, the cancer has not spread to other parts of the body

OR: The cancer has spread to lymph nodes around the major central airways while the tumor has grown into the mediastinum or other vital structures

OR: There are several nodules in different lobes of the same lung.

Stage IV: The tumor can be of any size and in any local lymph nodes, but it has spread to distant sites, such as to the opposite lung, other organs, lymph nodes outside of the lung, or bone. Cancers that cause (and are involved in) fluid buildup inside the lungs or around the heart (called "effusions") are also considered Stage IV.

SMALL CELL LUNG CANCER STAGING

Small cell lung cancer has a similar staging system as above, but doctors frequently use a simplified system that divides patients into two categories based on the type of treatment they are expected to receive:

Limited Stage: The primary tumor and lymph nodes are in a confined area of the chest that is amenable to radiation therapy, and there are no other sites of disease.

Extensive Stage: Cancer has spread to areas that cannot be encompassed with radiation or the cancer has spread to other parts of the body.

What types of blood tests and scans or treatments are necessary before deciding on a treatment strategy?

Once a complete and thorough staging of the tumor has been done as mentioned previously, there are several tests that need to be completed prior to initiating treatment. Blood tests such as a Complete Blood Count (CBC) and a Comprehensive Metabolic Panel (CMP) must be done. The CBC is used to determine baseline levels of white blood cells, red blood cells, and platelets. The CMP provides information about the electrolytes in the body and the function of the kidneys and liver. Baseline CT or PET/CT scans will be done, which can be used to determine how effectively the treatment is working in the future. Often, an MRI (Magnetic Resonance Imaging) of the brain will be done to ensure that there is no evidence of spread of cancer. If surgery is being considered, Pulmonary Function Tests (PFT) may be done to assess the capacity and function of the lungs. Finally, some treatment plans may require pretreatment with certain vitamins and steroids in order to decrease the incidence of side effects from chemotherapy.

Importantly, the Pathologist may perform a variety of tests on the tissue from the tumor biopsy. These tests will be used to determine if the cancer has certain characteristics like mutations that can help guide treatment with approved drugs or on clinical trials. EGFR mutations, EML4/ALK rearrangements and KRAS mutations, are a few examples. Scientists are continually developing new molecular treatments for the future (i.e. designer drugs).

What is the difference between metastatic and non-metastatic cancer? What is a metastasis?

Metastatic refers to a new colony of cancer cells that has spread to a different location than where the primary lung tumor started (i.e. lymph nodes or other organs). This often involves spread of cancer to the bone or to different organs in the body such as the liver or brain (distant metastases) and is usually no longer treatable by surgery or radiation for cure. Tumors that have only spread to adjacent lymph nodes (regional metastases) and not to other organs are still potentially curable. **Non metastatic** refers to cancer that is still localized in the lung and may be treatable

NURSE'S NOTE:

It is important to stop smoking both for health and healing. This can be challenging. Your nurse can help you find resources to help you meet the challenge.

with surgery or radiation alone, or some combination of chemotherapy, radiation, and surgery for cure.

Are there any screening tests for Lung Cancer?

Since lung cancer can develop without symptoms, most professional societies now recommend lung screening with a low-radiation CT scan of the chest in high risk individuals. This is based on the recent results of a national screening trial that showed a 20% reduction in lung cancer mortality with CT screening compared to conventional chest x-rays. High-risk individuals in this trial were defined as patients age 55-74 years old who had at least a 30 pack/year smoking history (1 pack per day for 30 years or equivalent), and if they were former smokers, they had to have quit within 15 years.

Because lung cancer screening is new, most hospitals haven't set up screening programs yet. You should expect these programs to be set up soon in your area.

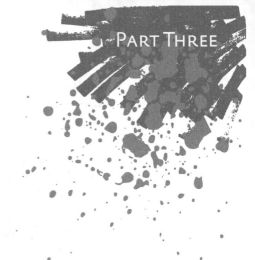
Will I Need Surgical Treatment?

How is a Thoracic Surgeon involved in the care of patients with Lung Cancer?

A general thoracic surgeon is a surgeon who specializes in non-cardiac diseases of the chest, with a particular focus in cancer surgery. However, the majority of lung cancer resections in the U.S. are performed by cardiac surgeons and cardiothoracic surgeons who operate on both the heart and the lungs, or by general surgeons who operate on all parts of the body. Nevertheless, most large cancer centers recognize the value in having dedicated thoracic surgeons who focus exclusively on cancers of the chest, as it allows the surgeons to be abreast of the latest developments and technology, as well as be an integral member of the multidisciplinary lung cancer team. Studies have shown that thoracic surgeons have better outcomes with lung cancer resections due to this sub-specialized focus.

The thoracic surgeon works very closely with his or her colleagues in medical oncology, radiation oncology, radiology, and pulmonology to coordinate multidisciplinary care. Consultation with a thoracic surgeon is critical in the evaluation of lung cancer for several reasons. First, the surgeon will be able to determine if resection is possible or not. Second, the surgeon can obtain a tissue diagnosis if needed. Third, the surgeon can determine if there has been any spread into the lymph nodes in the mediastinum or central chest compartment, which is a critical step in staging.

What are available options for biopsy?

From the outside of the body, a CT-guided needle biopsy can be performed by a radiologist to withdraw cells out of the tumor. This should be done with what is called a "core" needle so that sufficient tissue is obtained. From the inside of the body, a bronchoscopy can be performed, which is a fiber-optic endoscope (long, thin camera) that is passed into the airway to visualize the tumor directly (see pages 8-9, fig 2.2). A newer technology called electromagnetic navigational bronchoscopy allows the surgeon or pulmonologist to go out further in the lung field using special "GPS-like" technology. This allows for very precise biopsies with a lower risk of collapsing the lung than with CT guided needle biopsy. Finally, in some cases a surgical resection may be recommended as both a diagnostic and therapeutic procedure.

What tests help to decide if surgery is possible or necessary?

The two considerations that determine if cancer can be removed surgically are: 1) the extent of disease and 2) the patient's overall health.

In most cases, resectable (surgically removable) lung cancer must be localized to one side of the chest. Sometimes chemotherapy and/or radiation will be given prior to surgical resection if there has been spread into the lymph nodes of the mediastinum or central compartment of the chest. The extent of the disease is determined by CT and PET/CT scans, as well as by biopsy of the lymph nodes in the mediastinum. However, there are some cases where lung cancer can be resected even in stage IV disease, such as when there are limited metastases to the brain only. Therefore, the stage designation is not an automatic determination of how the tumor will be treated.

The patient's overall health is a very important consideration in determining the role of surgery. For some patients, any type of surgical resection would be too much physiologic stress on the body, making the risk of surgery too high. In other patients, the amount of lung tissue that can be removed is limited by emphysema or COPD (Chronic Obstructive Pulmonary Disease). Surgeons use cardiac stress tests, pulmonary function tests, and clinical judgment in assessing the safety of surgery for a given patient. Nowadays, patients who cannot tolerate surgery are considered for alternative treatments such as stereotactic body radiation (SBRT or sometimes called "radiosurgery") or destruction with thermal energy or freezing (radio frequency ablation or cryoablation, respectively).

How does the surgeon help in staging?

Determining the stage of lung cancer is critical in

the evaluation of a patient to ensure that the appropriate treatment is recommended. Distant spread of the cancer to sites outside of the chest is determined with a PET/CT scan and a brain MRI or CT scan. Additionally, the mediastinum or central compartment of the chest is a frequent site of lymph node metastases that has significant implications on treatment and prognosis. Unfortunately, radiographic scans such as a PET/CT scan are not 100% reliable in the assessment of these lymph nodes and a biopsy procedure is often required. Staging of the mediastinum is achieved by two techniques, both of which are very safe and can be done in the outpatient setting.

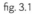 fig. 3.1

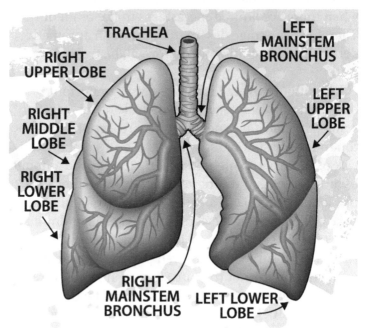

Lung anatomy

Cervical mediastinoscopy is the traditional method of sampling the lymph nodes in the mediastinum. This involves making a small 3 cm incision near the sternal notch (top of the breastbone) at the lower part of the neck. A small video camera is inserted into the incision and guided into the mediastinum alongside the windpipe to access the lymph nodes in the central part of the chest. Biopsies are directly obtained and sent for examination under a microscope.

A newer technique that is increasingly being used for biopsying these lymph nodes uses **endobronchial ultrasound or EBUS**. Usually done by either a thoracic surgeon or a pulmonologist, this does not require an incision and instead relies upon a special bronchoscope with an ultrasound probe at the tip. It is inserted through the mouth into the windpipe and the ultrasound is used to identify the lymph nodes located adjacent to the wall of the airway. Under ultra-

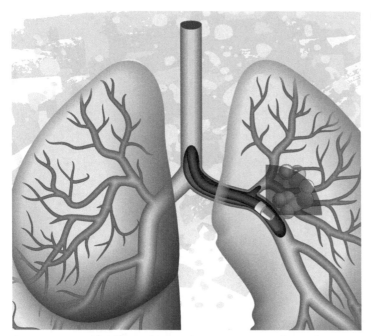

fig. 3.2

Lung anatomy details can be seen by a camera put down the throat and into the bronchus, This camera has an ultrasound and can measure, view, and help to biopsy tumors or lymph nodes. It is called "endobronchial ultrasound" (EBUS).

sound guidance, a needle is passed through the scope into the lymph node to suction out some of the tissue, which is then sent for microscopic evaluation.

What types of surgery are there? (i.e., lobectomy, pneumonectomy, wedge resection, etc.)

A person's lungs are comprised of 3 lobes on the right side (upper, middle, and lower) and 2 lobes on the left side (upper and middle)*(see fig. 3.1)*. A lobe is an anatomic component of the lung that has its own blood supply and airway. The lobe can be further comprised of segments. The extent of resection necessary depends on the extent of the tumor as well as the ability of the patient to tolerate lung removal.

A *pneumonectomy* is removal of the entire lung on one side of the chest. These operations are usually required for tumors that are centrally located where the vessels and airways to the lobes originate. Typically, the tumor encroaches on all of the lobes, requiring resection of the whole lung.

A *lobectomy* is removal of one lobe of the lung. This is the standard method of resection for most cancers. Studies have shown that local recurrence is decreased when a lobectomy is performed compared to lesser resections.

A *segmentectomy* is removal of one or more segments from a lobe and sparing the rest of the segments. These resections are limited to tumors that are peripheral and small, generally less than 2 cm.

A *wedge resection* is simply resecting the tumor with a margin of surrounding lung regardless of the segmental anatomy. Similar to a segmentectomy, this type of resection is limited to tumors that are peripheral and small.

* Your surgeon will discuss with you what the best type of operation is for your situation.

What technologies are available in this modern era to improve surgery and healing?

The traditional method of performing a lung resection has been with a **thoracotomy**. This incision involves making a 15-20 cm incision along the side of the chest and spreading the ribs apart to enter the chest.

Over the past 20 years, surgeons have been relying more on **thoracoscopic or VATS (video-assisted thoracoscopic surgery)** to perform surgery. This is a minimally invasive operation that is analogous to laparoscopic surgery in the abdomen. It involves making 3 or 4 small incisions between the ribs through which a video camera and small instruments are used to perform the operation. Most importantly, there should be no spreading or breaking of the ribs during a VATS procedure.

Despite the advantages of VATS procedures, most lung resections in the United States are still done with a thoracotomy due to ergonomic issues and technical challenges of working with long, straight instruments through tiny incisions in the chest wall. As a result, some surgeons are now using **robotic surgery** to overcome these problems. Similar to VATS, small incisions are made without rib spreading, through which a special camera allows the surgeon to see in 3-D, and tiny wristed robotic instruments allow precise surgery that replicates the surgeon's hands and wrists inside the rigid chest cavity.

NURSE'S NOTE:

Any surgical procedure has the chance for infection. Signs may be fever, redness, chills, pain, swelling, and/ or warmth of the area. Let your nurse know if you experience any of these symptoms.

Minimally invasive techniques with either VATS or robotic techniques have revolutionized lung cancer surgery and allow far faster recovery than with a thoracotomy, and with less pain.

fig. 3.3

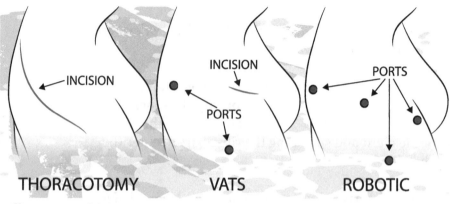

Different types of chest incisions

What types of blood tests and scans are necessary before deciding on a final treatment strategy?

Recent imaging is critical to assess the size and location of the tumor. This typically entails a CT scan and/or PET/CT scan within 4-6 weeks of the planned treatment. A PET/CT will give information about metastatic spread to other parts of the body, such as the adrenal glands, liver, or bone. A separate brain MRI or CT is often done to determine if there are metastases to the brain, as a PET/CT usually cannot give reliable information for this part of the body.

An evaluation for lung resection will also include a cardiac stress test and a pulmonary function test to determine the health of the patient and the ability to undergo major thoracic surgery. There are several types of cardiac stress tests, and the specific one is usually chosen by local preference. A pulmonary function test is used to measure the lung capacity and function to ensure that the lungs have enough reserve to allow for the planned resection.

All surgical procedures will require a basic blood test, including tests that test the clotting ability of the blood. There are no routine blood tests at the current time that aid clinicians with decision-making for lung cancer treatment, although several are currently being investigated.

What is the difference between metastatic and non-metastatic cancer? What is a metastasis and is surgery an option for metastatic disease?

Metastasis means that a focus of cancer has spread outside of its primary site of origin. There are different degrees of metastases, so there is no single treatment plan for metastases in general. If metastases occurred to the lymph nodes, treatment will depend on where the lymph nodes are located, and in some cases, how many nodes are involved. Sometimes lymph node metastases prevent surgical resection, and other times it does not. If metastases have occurred outside of the chest or to the opposite side of the chest, this usually means surgery is not an option, but again there are exceptions. For example, brain metastases are often treated with surgery and followed by lung resection. Assessment of metastases and making a treatment plan is often not straightforward or rigid, especially since every patient is unique, which highlights the value of being assessed by a multidisciplinary team of cancer experts.

How do you prepare patients for surgery (tests)?

Imaging studies such as a CT scan are usually

updated if they are older than 4-6 weeks to minimize the chance of any unexpected finding in the operating room. In addition, a cardiac stress test is often done to ensure the patient's heart is healthy enough to undergo surgery. Pulmonary function tests will determine if there is sufficient lung reserve to undergo the planned resection.

Self preparation for surgery is very important for patients. It is critical that patients maintain a positive outlook, walk daily, and maintain a healthy diet. A patient's mental outlook and physical conditioning will significantly impact the recovery process.

What will happen on the day of surgery?

Most patients are instructed to arrive at the hospital approximately 2 hours prior to their scheduled operation. They should not to eat or drink anything after midnight the night before the operation, with the exception of critical medications that are specified by the surgeon or anesthesiologist. Typically, all of the necessary pre-operative tests have been reviewed prior to the day of surgery, so there is not a lot of testing (and potential for surprises) on the day of surgery. The patient will have a chance to meet the operating room nurse, anesthesia team, and surgical team prior to going into the operating room. An IV will be started and some additional paperwork will be completed. Most hospitals require that the side of surgery (left or right) be marked with a permanent marker by the surgical team prior to entering the operating room. Nurses may ask the patient to verify that they understand the procedure or explain what is being done – this is not asked because there is confusion but to ensure that the patient is well-informed and educated about the planned operation.

Surgical Recovery

The patient's recovery is dependent on the type of operation that is performed. A minimally invasive lobectomy with either robotic or VATS techniques will allow much faster recovery than with a traditional thoracotomy incision. A minimally invasive lobectomy will require 2-4 days in the hospital to recover, compared to 6-10 days with a thoracotomy. With either a minimally invasive or open operation, most patients spend the first night in the ICU or step down unit, and the remainder of the hospital stay is on the surgical ward.

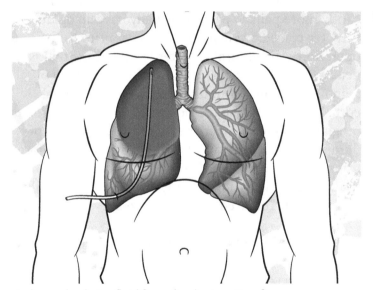

fig. 3.4

A chest tube drains fluid from the chest cavity after surgery.

When the patient awakens from surgery there will usually be a **chest tube**, which is a soft plastic tube that drains the chest in the postoperative setting. This tube is placed on suction and remains in place until the lung is re-inflated, at which point it is removed prior to going home. The day after surgery most patients are able to get out of bed, sit in a chair, and walk around the hallway. Patients are also able to eat starting on the first postoperative day.

Pain is dependent on the type of surgery performed and, of course, ultimately can be very different for each person. Nevertheless, minimally invasive operations result in significantly less pain than with an open thoracotomy. Following a robotic or VATS operation, postoperative pain is controlled with oral pain pills with the occasional need for intravenous medications during the first day or two. **Oral pain pills** are typically continued on an as-needed basis for a week or two. With a thoracotomy, there is significantly more pain so patients usually have an epidural catheter placed by an anesthesiologist prior to the operation. An epidural catheter is a tiny tube that is inserted into the back and allows direct delivery of pain medications around the outside of the spinal cord. This is the same method used for pain control in pregnant women who are delivering a baby. The epidural catheter is typically used for several days before transitioning to oral and intravenous pain medications. Following a thoracotomy, use of oral pain pills is commonly required for several weeks.

Possible Post-surgery Complications

Patients recover earlier if they limit their time in bed and increase their time spent upright and walking. This helps re-inflate lungs that may have collapsed due to the operation. This can sometimes lead to a fever and some cases can result in **pneumonia**. To further encourage deep breathing, many hospitals provide patients with a **spirometer**, which is small plastic device that allows breathing exercises to be performed while in bed or in a chair.

In some instances, a small air leak may persist from the remaining lung. This can occur as the resected lung is separated from the remaining lung. It will almost always resolve with time.

Atrial fibrillation is another relatively common issue that can arise following surgery. This is an irregular, fast heart rate that is commonly observed following operations in the chest. When it occurs, it is controlled with medications, and rarely requires further intervention. The risk of developing atrial fibrillation is greatest in the immediate post-operative period. Many surgeons routinely administer medications to patients in the recovery period to decrease the chance of atrial fibrillation.

As with any other type of major surgery, risks of other complications include bleeding, infection, stroke, heart attack, and death. Lobectomy in high-volume centers is safe, with a mortality rate of approximately 1-2%.

Follow-up and Complementary Therapy

How often is follow-up recommended and what types of blood tests, scans, and other symptoms are watched for in the future? Is any physical therapy, respiratory therapy, or other alternative or complementary treatments recommended?

Following discharge from the hospital after surgery, patients will typically see the surgeon one or two times during the first month. Afterwards, patients are placed into surveillance to detect any recurrence that could develop. In coordination with the patient's oncologist, patients are usually followed with CT scans of the chest every 3-4 months initially, and then usually increased to every 6-12 months after the first 3 years. Since the greatest risk of recurrence is within the first 3 years after surgery, this is the time period of most intense surveillance. There is no standardized blood test that is used for lung cancer follow up at this time, although several are being investigated.

Formal physical therapy is usually not necessary after surgery, especially with a minimally invasive operation. However, patients are encouraged to walk every day and gradually get back into exercising. Physical healing will occur quite rapidly but fatigue can linger, especially if chemotherapy or radiation is included in one's treatment. This lack of energy is expected and can last for a few months before patients feel completely back to normal.

Complementary treatments are acceptable if they do not interfere with other medically indicated treatment. It is very important that if such treatments are pursued that patients communicate with their regular physicians to ensure that there will be no issues or harmful interactions with medications.

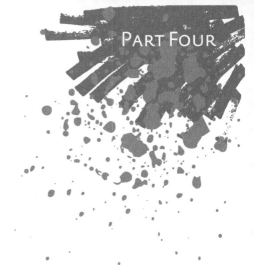

PART FOUR

What Is Radiation Therapy?

Radiation Therapy

Radiation therapy, or radiotherapy, is a cancer treatment that uses high dose x-rays directed at a target or tumor to kill cancer cells. It is a local treatment, meaning it treats only those tissues at which it is aimed or directed. The x-rays pass through the body and do not deposit or remain in the patient's body tissues.

The effect of x-rays on the tumor cell is to damage the cell, and potentially, to cause the tumor or mass to shrink or disappear entirely. Likewise, radiation therapy can cause changes to normal, healthy tissues that surround the targeted area of the body. The effect of radiation on normal tissues is what leads to side effects.

fig. 4.1

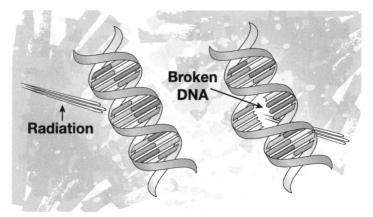

Radiation works by causing breaks in the DNA strands within cancer cells. This leads to cancer cell death.

Radiotherapy can be given a number of ways, including externally (outside the body), via x-rays that are emitted from large treatment machines, or internally (inside the body), via specially designed applicators or devices that hold a source of radiation within a body site or cavity. Different forms of radiotherapy are used depending on the target, part of the body and other technical considerations. The majority of cancer patients who receive radiation treatments receive the external type.

Radiation therapy is used extensively in lung cancer. Additionally, it is a main component of treating many other cancers including those of the breast, prostate, rectum, head and neck region, and brain. Radiation therapy will often be used in addition to (either before or following) surgery. Radiation therapy can be given following chemotherapy (sequentially), as in women being treated for breast cancer, or can be given simultaneously (concurrently, or at the same time) to patients with lung, head and neck, and rectal cancers. The side effects of any cancer treatment largely depend on the treatment combinations that are given.

Potential side effects of treatment for lung cancer will typically be worse in those that receive a combination of radiation and chemotherapy at the same time.

The use of radiation therapy for patients with lung cancer is largely dependent on the stage (location and extent) of the cancer and the health of the patient. Surgical resection of lung cancer, if possible, is recognized as the best chance for cure in patients suffering from the illness. However, not all patients are a candidate for surgical removal because of their health or because the cancer is too large, extensive, or positioned in a part of the body that makes it too difficult to remove. Radiation therapy often serves as an alternative.

Radiation therapy for lung cancer can be given with the goal to destroy the cancer in an effort to cure the disease. This approach would be considered **definitive** or **curative** and depending on the situation might require the additional use of chemotherapy. Some patients with poor health or widely advanced (metastatic) disease, may receive radiotherapy with a goal to help relieve symptoms (such as cough, bleeding, shortness of breath, pain) rather than to cure the cancer. This approach is considered **palliative** (for comfort only) and would typically be completed without chemotherapy at the same time. The length of time of your radiation therapy course will depend on the goal of therapy, stage of disease and overall treatment plan.

Radiation Therapy for Lung Cancer

The use of radiotherapy in lung cancer is very common and depends largely on the location and extent of the cancer. Prior to starting a course of radiotherapy, it is common for a patient to have a number of

NURSE'S NOTE:

Depending upon the goals of treatment, radiation courses can range from 1–7 weeks.

studies and scans performed, in addition to a physical examination, to aid in determining the site (or target) for treatment. Common scans include computed-tomography (or CT) of the chest, bone scan, positron-emission tomography (or PET), head CT or magnetic resonance imaging (MRI), among others specific to your situation. Standard blood examinations including blood count and chemistries are commonly obtained too. Often, those images from these tests will be used by your physician to create your radiation treatment plan.

fig. 4.2

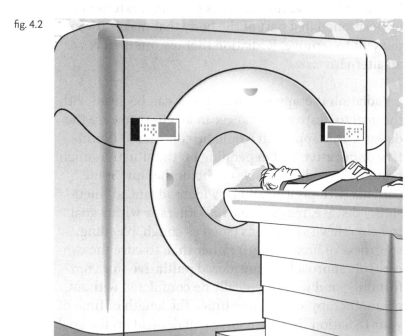

CT scans allow your doctors to map out the extent of the cancer spread.

In lung cancer, internal delivery of radiation therapy is rarely used. More commonly, external x-rays are delivered to the target or tumor by special machines that are programmed to deliver the treatment (Linear Accelerators). The treatment is a local treatment,

fig. 4.3

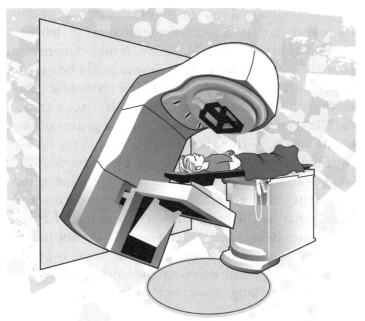

The most common machine used for radiation treatment is called a Linear Accelerator.

meaning it effects only those tissues it is aimed at, but is also "conformal", meaning the treatment x-rays are shaped to match the shape and position of the target or tumor. Often, multiple beams of x-rays will be used during each radiation treatment to deliver the radiotherapy. Using multiple beams that shape the x-ray to match the target is called 3-D conformal radiotherapy (3DCRT). New technologies, in addition to shaping the x-rays, allow for the strength of the x-ray to be changed or modulated during treatment delivery in an effort to avoid or spare normal tissues that are frequently found next to the target or tumor. This treatment is called intensity-modulated radiotherapy or IMRT. Your treating physician will determine the best way to plan and deliver your treatment based on the information that has been gathered since your cancer diagnosis.

NURSE'S NOTE:

New radiation machines allow the beams to be aimed precisely every day at internal locations.

NURSE'S NOTE:

Ask about the short and long-term effects of treatment. Some treatments have effects that can be noticed months or years later.

Given the natural movement of the lungs, your doctor may recommend technologies that aid in delivering radiation to targets that move. A four-dimensional computed tomography (4DCT) scan might be obtained during the mapping/planning session (see the section on "Simulation", page 36). A 4DCT scan essentially takes a CT image during multiple phases of the breathing cycle. This allows your doctor to see how your tumor moves with breathing. Other possible ways to account for motion include respiration-gated techniques (delivering the treatment only during a specific part of the breathing cycle), or breath hold techniques (where they teach you to hold your breath to minimize motion). Sometimes a device may be used to apply pressure to your abdomen in order to help minimize lung movement during treatment.

Modern radiotherapy methods for treating lung cancers are currently being investigated and may be used to treat your cancer. Image guided radiation therapy (IGRT) is the process of obtaining frequent (often daily) images to help position the tumor correctly. Sometimes a CT scan or radiograph may be acquired during treatment for use in IGRT. Stereotactic Body Radiotherapy (or SBRT) is a specialized form of 3DCRT or IMRT where a tumor is targeted by multiple angles in only a few (1-5) very intense (much higher than standard daily) doses. By targeting a single target with 10 or more x-rays or treatment fields, the normal tissues that surround the tumor will receive very little radiation dose. However, at the center of where those 10 or more beams intersect, or meet, the radiation dose is quite high and powerful. This technique, SBRT, is used primarily for patients with small tumors who are not eligible for surgical removal.

fig. 4.4

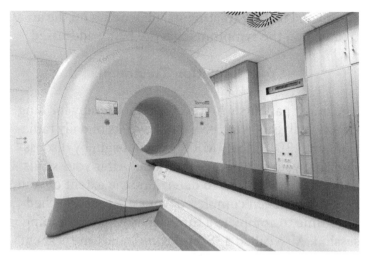

Tomotherapy (Accuray) is a modern radiotherapy treatment machine which has the capability of detailed daily imaging of a patients anatomy before treatment. This allows for refined treatment of the cancer and further protection of surrounding normal organs.

Additionally, proton beam therapy (PBT) is being investigated as an alternative to the standard x-ray approach. Although similar in its impact on normal and cancerous tissues, PBT has the possible advantage of reducing effects on the normal, surrounding organs because of its unique characteristics. PBT is not commonly available and is currently only being offered at a few, highly specialized centers worldwide and is being heavily studied by research groups.

The total length of your course or treatment of radiation therapy depends on the type of radiation used, intent or goal of treatment as well as some other factors. When SBRT is used, the total treatment is usually 3 to 5 times over 1 to 2 ½ weeks. When a standard course of radiation is delivered for more advanced lung cancers (either with or without chemotherapy) the total treatment course can be 30 to 35 treatments over 6 to 7 weeks. If you are receiving palliative radiation (to help with or prevent symptoms), that can be completed in 1-20 treatments, depending on the area treated and the symptoms that are being addressed.

Your Radiation Treatments

As most patients who receive radiotherapy for lung cancer will usually receive 6 to 7 weeks of daily radiation, with 3DCRT or IMRT, we will begin by discussing what your experience might be. After your scans and other evaluations to determine the extent of your cancer have been completed, your doctor will schedule a time to complete a tumor mapping or planning session. Also called a "**Simulation**", this time is spent in determining the position you will be treated in everyday, obtaining any needed scans, placing marks (possibly with permanent tattoos) on your skin and preparing any other items necessary to start your radiotherapy. It commonly will take 40 to 60 minutes. During the session, any special shaping pillows, beanbags or special molding devices will be created to fit to your body and assist in positioning you for each of your treatments. Usually, there is no requirement to fast or make any other special preparations for this time. If your doctor does require you to take a special medication, drink or swallow something before planning or treatments, or other special preparation methods, they will notify you.

After the simulation or planning session is complete, your physician and his or her team of staff will begin to take all of the information gathered and will develop a treatment plan specific to your cancer and your body. Your physician and staff use highly specialized computers to develop the treatment plans. This process may take several days to complete. Once they have created an optimized treatment plan they will arrange for your treatments to start.

NURSE'S NOTE:

It is important that you keep all of your appointments for radiation treatment for optimal results. If you miss a session, it may be added to the end of treatment or as a second treatment on another day if you choose.

When your treatments begin, you will find that most days are quite similar. The radiotherapy staff (radiation therapists) will escort you into the treatment room. They may have you change into a gown either before or after entering the room. Once you have changed and are in the room, they will utilize the devices created at your planning session on the treatment table and will have you get on the table and recreate that position that was determined at the planning time. You will be positioned on the table and they will begin the process of moving the table and machine to align the marks on your skin with special light and lasers in the room (these are not the x-rays). This can sometimes take a few minutes. After you are positioned, they will ask that you remain still for the remainder of the treatment. Typically, your treatment will take 5 to 20 minutes to deliver. They will exit the room to deliver the treatment. You can communicate with the staff easily as the treatment room is connected to the control area by two-way microphones and speakers. Furthermore, they will monitor or watch you as you have your treatment through a number of cameras that are positioned throughout the treatment room.

During your treatment, it is important that you remain as still as reasonably possible. If you develop an issue with being still, then the staff may have to stop the treatment and/or reposition you prior to completing the treatment for that day. As the x-rays are delivered you will not feel, smell, or sense anything. The machine does make different noises as it functions, but this should not impact you. You should not expect to feel any burning, itching, or other irritations as the treatment is being delivered. Once the treatment for that day is completed, the staff will enter the room once again, rotate the machinery and table back to their starting position, and allow you to get off the table and exit the room and get dressed. When you leave, there will be no radiation left in you and you are not a danger to other people.

During the course of your therapy, your physician and staff will meet with you periodically to discuss the progress of your treatment, your health, and any side effects you may be experiencing. Typically, these visits are scheduled once a week and will immediately follow or precede your treatment that day. However, if you are feeling poorly, have questions, or are concerned about any new issues, you should feel free to discuss this with the staff when you arrive for your daily treatment.

Alternatively, those patients who will receive SBRT as their treatment should expect to have a little different experience then that described. The primary difference is the length of therapy. First, SBRT is delivered in 3 to 5 treatments over 1 to 4 ½ weeks, rather than over six to seven weeks as described. Second, the daily treatment could take as long as 60 minutes or more to deliver (depending on the complexity), rather than the 15 minutes described above for the conventional approach of radiation therapy. It is important that you provide feedback to your treatment team during your planning and simulation to ensure your maximum comfort; the position you are in at planning will be your treatment position. If this is hard or uncomfortable in any way, it will make it all the more difficult to remain as still as possible for the SBRT treatment time.

Similar to the conventional approach, when you arrive for your SBRT you will be escorted to the treatment room and will change into a hospital gown.

fig. 4.5

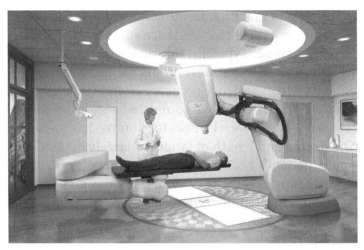

The CyberKnife system (Accuray) is a type of radiation machine designed for pin-point tracking and robotic delivery of focused radiation. This machine can physically track and treat tumors in the lung as they are moving during breathing motion.

The staff will assist you in getting positioned in your treatment pillow or positioning device and will then perform a series of movements, with you on the treatment table, to position you correctly. Again, it is extremely important you **remain as still as possible** for the entire time you are on the treatment table. You should feel welcome to relax and even take a nap if you wish during this time. If the staff or your physician wish you to prepare for your SBRT in a specific way (take an anti-nausea pill before treatment, not eat for a certain period of time preceding treatment, etc.), they will let you know at the time of your planning so you can come prepared on the first day of your radiation therapy.

Side Effects of Radiation Therapy

The side effects that develop during and following a course of radiotherapy largely depend on the location and extent of treatment. Many patients, regardless of the type of radiation treatment and the length of therapy can expect to experience some level of **tiredness or fatigue**. Typically, this tiredness is not overwhelming or debilitating, but it is noticeable. Many patients will experience recovery from this fatigue once the treatments have completed and sufficient recovery time (several weeks to months) has passed. The degree and length of fatigue is largely dependent on the patient's health status at the time of starting radiotherapy, whether chemotherapy was given with the radiation treatments, and the severity of side effects that developed before completing the course of radiotherapy.

Another common side effect that develops with radiotherapy for lung cancer is **swallowing pain and difficulty** (esophagitis or irritation of the esophagus or "food pipe"). Again, the severity and duration of this side effect is highly variable and depends on the location of your tumor, whether you receive chemotherapy, and the length of your treatment course. The swallowing difficulty can be something as minor as a "lump-sensation" in the throat with swallowing, to a severe inability to swallow food, liquids, or even your own phlegm (spit). Pain can also develop and is typically worsened by trying to swallow. Your physician will be able to provide or prescribe any number of courses of action or medications to assist with the discomfort and dysfunction. Ultimately, a few patients will not be able to swallow for an extended period of time and therefore a feeding tube will be need to be placed and used as a means of food and nutrition. Fortunately, the majority of patients with swallowing pain and dysfunction will experience improvement in a couple of weeks to months after treatments are completed and they have an opportunity to heal.

Patients undergoing radiation treatment can experience **irritation, pain, and peeling of the skin**. Some changes are subtle and are only some slight reddening. Some skin changes are more obvious and occur with pain, blistering, itching and discomfort. The severity of skin reaction is again variable and many patients experience no skin change at all, even after 7 weeks of treatment. Your physician and treatment team will regularly check your skin and will monitor any changes, offering suggestions for skin care when needed. Fortunately, most skin changes will improve within days to weeks once the treatment has completed.

Radiation treatments can adversely impact the normal lung that surrounds the tumor or cancer target. During your course of treatment, any radiation-related lung injury often shows itself as increasing phlegm production, increased cough, and maybe heavy breathing (feeling short of air). However, many patients who have had a decline in lung function or severe cough may experience an improvement in their breathing or cough during their course of radiotherapy as the tumor shrinks and the affected lung begins to move air once again. Any cough, phlegm issues, or other breathing difficulties should be discussed with your physician and treatment team. In some patients, a month following radiation treatment or as long as 6 to 12 months later, progressive shortness of breath, cough and fever can develop; similar to developing a pneumonia. Your physician should be notified of these changes and an evaluation could reveal the symptoms. Some patients will experience radiation pneumonitis (an inflammation of the lung) caused by the course of radiotherapy, that mimics pneumonia, but is treated quite differently. Fortunately, many patients can be treated readily with anti-inflammatories or with steroids for this and will experience a recovery of lung function.

Rarely, radiation treatments can cause injury to other organs including the heart, spinal cord, chest wall (muscles and ribs), or blood vessels that will cause symptoms. Radiation-related heart injury often results from direct x-rays to the heart and can cause a heart pump dysfunction or coronary artery disease (many years later). Spinal cord injury could lead to pain, weakness or even complete paralysis (extremely rare). Damage caused by radiation to the muscles or ribs of the chest wall or to major blood vessels could result in weakening of the chest wall structure, pain, and dysfunction. The esophagus (food pipe) can develop scar tissue or become narrowed. This may require a dilation or stretching procedure. Fortunately, these injuries are quite rare and do not commonly impair an individual following radiotherapy.

Following Radiation Treatments

Once you have successfully completed your course of radiation therapy, your physician will arrange for you to return and discuss your recovery and to assess your cancer's response to the treatments. Commonly, you can expect to return the first time, following radiotherapy, in 2 to 8 weeks. At that point, your physician will decide when the appropriate time should be to get images (PET/CT) to assess the response should be and to assist you with any ongoing issues that may have developed owing to side effects from the radiotherapy. Most patients can expect to visit with their cancer doctors fairly regularly that first year after treatments are concluded, sometimes as often as every month, but usually every 3-6 months. Scans are typically performed every 3 to 6 months to check on the status of your normal tissues but also to check the response of the lung cancer and see if there are any signs of new, recurrent or persistent disease.

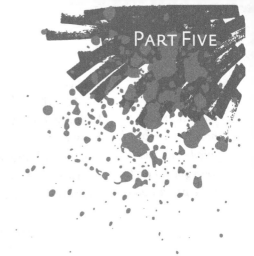

PART FIVE

What Are Chemotherapy And Biotherapy Treatment?

Lung cancer patients are treated by a multidisciplinary team of doctors that includes Medical Oncologists, Thoracic Surgeons, Radiation Oncologists, Pulmonologists, and Radiologists. Medical Oncologists are responsible for deciding which drugs, if any, are appropriate to treat the cancer and for the safe administration of that therapy. In some stages of lung cancer, chemotherapy is given with radiation therapy (chemo-radiation) or after surgery has been done (adjuvant chemotherapy). Chemotherapy means "chemical or drug" therapy. Chemotherapy is considered a **systemic** therapy (treats the whole body). These are medicines that are either taken orally or administered

NURSE'S NOTE:

Make sure you have a friend or family member with you for visits to help take notes.

intravenously (through the veins) that kill cancer cells or stop them from growing. They travel through the bloodstream to nearly all parts of the body. Therefore, they can treat cancer cells where they started or any cells that have already spread (metastasized). Chemotherapy can be used in combination with local therapies (radiation, surgery) or alone.

Most chemotherapies are given via an intravenous (IV) infusion and would require an IV start each time. Also some chemotherapies cause irritation to the small veins in the arms. To make the administration more streamlined and easier on the patient, an indwelling IV line (port or portacath) will often be used. This is a catheter device with a reservoir that is placed under the skin that connects into a major blood vessel. These are usually placed by a surgeon or an interventional radiologist in the upper chest. This allows easy IV access by inserting a needle through the skin into the reservoir. This is called "accessing" the port. This can be used for other IV medication, hydration, or drawing blood. This minimizes the number of "IV needle sticks" a patient needs to have. Ports need to be kept clean and will need to be "flushed" with saline and heparin (keeps it from clotting) every 4-6 weeks. Some ports are put in the arm.

NURSE'S NOTE:

Most facilities offer a chemo class prior to you starting therapy. This is a great way to learn about the drug you will be given and specific side effects it may have.

What are the differences between "curative" and "palliative" therapy?

Curative therapy is aimed at eliminating all traces of the cancer. Depending on the stage of the cancer, this can involve a combination of chemotherapy, radiation therapy, and surgery. Curative therapy is the goal for many patients with non-metastatic cancer. These are usually patients whose lung cancer has been staged from stage I to stage III.

Metastatic cancer patients are treated with palliative therapy. This is therapy aimed at alleviating the patient's symptoms from cancer and importantly, improving the patient's length and quality of life. Palliative therapy is not curative. Palliative therapy usually consists of targeted drugs, chemotherapy and/or radiation therapy. **New chemotherapy and targeted drugs are extending the life of patients with lung cancer more than ever before and promising new drugs are in clinical trials**.

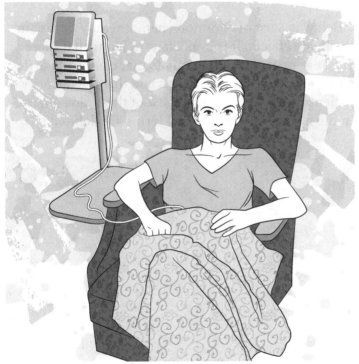

fig. 5.1

During IV (intravenous) Chemotherapy, you will be monitored while relaxing in a comfortable chair for a couple of hours with the chemotherapy being infused into your bloodstream.

What are the common chemotherapy treatments for lung cancer? When are they utilized, what is the duration of use, and what are the common side

effects? What are the common treatments for these side effects?

Chemotherapy agents are often given in combinations known as "**doublets**" or "**triplets**". In metastatic disease, after patients have received four to six cycles (courses) of chemotherapy they may be switched to **maintenance therapy** with a single chemotherapy drug. A new standard of care is to offer targeted drugs to treat a patient's lung cancer based on the results of specific mutation (abnormal cells) testing.

Below is a list of common chemotherapy drugs and their side effects. It is important to know that there are treatments and adjustments that can be made if a patient experiences side effects and that the majority of patients do not experience most of these side effects. In the next table, the medical terms are defined.

Drug Name	Alternate Names	Common Side Effects
Bevacizumab	Avastin	GI perforation, poor wound healing, blood clots, high blood pressure, protein in the urine, nose bleeds, bleeding
Carboplatin	Paraplatin	Myelosuppression, hypersensitivity reactions, neuropathy
Cisplatin	CDDP / Platinol	Nausea, vomiting, nephropathy, neuropathy, myelosuppression, ototoxicity
Crizotinib	Xalkori	Visual disturbances, rash, diarrhea, nausea/vomiting, fluid retention
Docetaxel	Taxotere	Hypersensitivity, myelosuppression, fluid retention,

		alopecia, neuropathy
Erlotinib	Tarceva	Rash, diarrhea
Etoposide	VP-16, Toposar, Vepsid	Myelosuppression, alopecia, mucositis, hypotension
Gemcitabine	Gemzar	Myelosuppression, flu like symptoms, rash, alopecia
Irinotecan	CPT-11, Camptosar	Diarrhea, myelosuppression, liver dysfunction, fever, chills, alopecia
Paclitaxel	Taxol	Myelosuppression, neuropathy, myalgia, alopecia, hypersensitivity
Pemetrexed	Alimta	Myelosuppression, fatigue, rash, nausea/vomiting, diarrhea
Topotecan	Hycamtin	Myelosuppression, nausea/vomiting, alopecia
Vinorelbine	Navelbine	Myelosuppression, liver dysfunction, neuropathy, constipation, alopecia

Side Effect	Definition
Alopecia	Hair loss
Hypersensitivity	Allergic reaction
Mucositis	Mouth sores
Myalgia	Muscle aches
Myelosuppression	Decrease in blood counts such as white blood cells, red blood cells, or platelets
Nephropathy	Kidney damage, decline in kidney function

Neuropathy	Damage to nerves causing numbness, tingling
Ototoxicity	Hearing loss, ringing in the ears

fig. 5.2

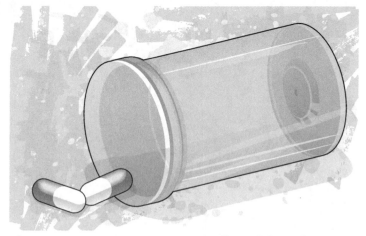

There are many new ways to treat side effects of chemotherapy that greatly lessen the severity experienced.

Medical Oncologists have an array of **supportive medications** that can be used to alleviate side effects. In cases where there are no medications to combat side effects, dose adjustments to the medications can be made by the doctor. Some of the commonly used supportive medications are as follows:

Drug Name	Alternate Names	Use
Ondansetron	Zofran	Nausea and vomiting
Granisetron	Kytril	Nausea and vomiting
Metoclopramide	Reglan	Nausea and vomiting
Aprepitant	Emend	Nausea and vomiting

Prochlorperazine	Compazine	Nausea and vomiting
Lorazepam	Ativan	Anxiety, nausea/vomiting
Dexamethasone	Decadron	Nausea/vomiting, hypersensitivity
Filgrastim	Neupogen	Increase blood counts to combat myelosuppression
Pegfilgrastim	Neulasta	Increase blood counts to combat myelosuppression
Diphenhydramine	Benadryl	Hypersensitivity
Ranitidine	Zantac	Nausea
Cobalamin	Vitamin B12	Myelosuppression
Folic Acid	Folate	Myelosuppression
Viscous Lidocaine	Lidocaine	Mucositis
Phenergan	Promethazine	Nausea and vomiting
Aloxi	Palonosetron	Nausea and vomiting
Pepcid	Famotidine	Nausea and vomiting
Doxycycline	Doxycycline	Rash
Minocycline	Minocycline	Rash
Clindamycin	Clindamycin ointment	Rash

What will the patient experience in the chemotherapy room when they receive treatment? How can they prepare and what should they expect?

Chemotherapy is usually given in an outpatient

clinic called an infusion center. In preparation for chemotherapy, the patient should take all pre medications as prescribed by their doctor.

On the day of chemotherapy, the patient will check in with the nurse or the port will be accessed in the infusion center and will be assigned a bed or chair where they will receive the chemotherapy. The nurse will then check the chemotherapy orders and the patient's blood test results to ensure that chemotherapy is safe to give on that day.

An intravenous line (IV line) will be started by the nurse and then a combination of hydration and/or the supportive medications previously mentioned will be given to minimize and/or prevent some side effects of chemotherapy. The chemotherapy drugs that have been ordered will then be administered over the course of several hours.

Upon completion of the chemotherapy, the nurse will disconnect the tubing and remove the IV (or de-access the port) line and the patient will be given an appointment for their next dose of chemotherapy. They should also have supportive medications to be taken at home in case they experience side effects.

What other therapies are available for the treatment of metastatic lung cancer? What are their side effects and advantages?

At many larger treatment centers, as an alternative to standard chemotherapy or when chemotherapy does not work to combat the lung cancer, patients may be offered the opportunity to participate in **clinical trials (research studies)**. Clinical trials involve the use of combinations of approved drugs in new ways or the administration of newly developed drugs that have not yet been approved by the U.S. Food and Drug Administration. If a Medical Oncologist thinks that a patient is a good candidate for a clinical trial and would benefit from participating, they will explain the rationale of the trial along with the risks, benefits, and alternatives to the patient and ask the patient to sign an informed consent document. The patient will then undergo whatever testing needs to be done to complete the enrollment process and initiate treatment under the clinical trial.

What can be done to strengthen bones?

Metastatic lung cancer often spreads to distant areas of the body, such as the brain and the bones. Brain metastases can cause a variety of symptoms including headaches, blurry vision, dizziness, weakness, and numbness. Bone metastases can cause bone pain and fractures. These types of metastases can often be treated with radiation therapy to improve symptoms (see chapter 4).

Patients with bone metastases are at risk for fractures. A Medical Oncologist may prescribe medications called Zoledronic Acid (Zometa) or Denosumab (Xgeva) to decrease the risk of fractures. Possible side effects of these medications include kidney dysfunction, low blood calcium levels and very rarely, damage

NURSE'S NOTE:
No one can tell you how you should feel. Just be in touch with your feelings and don't be afraid to ask for help.

NURSE'S NOTE:
Good dental hygiene is important during treatment. Use a soft, non-abrasive toothpaste and consult your dentist if any problems arise. Let your dentist know you are undergoing treatment for cancer.

to the bones of the jaw (osteonecrosis). If a patient is receiving these medications the physician should be made aware if any dental work is planned as this increases the risk of osteonecrosis (breakdown of the bone) of the jaw.

How often is follow-up recommended and what types of blood tests, scans, and other symptoms are watched for in the future? Are other therapies recommended like physical therapy, respiratory therapy, or other alternative or complementary treatments?

The follow-up during cancer therapy varies for each patient. It depends on the chemotherapy combination that the patient is receiving, the patient's response to treatment, and the symptoms that the patient is having. In general patients should be seen by their Medical Oncologist prior to each cycle of chemotherapy to assess symptoms and to check blood tests to monitor for any organ function abnormality or for low blood counts. PET/CT scans are typically done after every two or three therapy cycles to assess the cancer's response to chemotherapy.

NURSE'S NOTE:

Mental health professionals are not just available for the patient, they can help families gain coping skills as well.

Physical therapy and respiratory therapy are not routinely recommended, but may be quite helpful if the patient has specific symptoms. If the patient is experiencing difficulty with performing everyday tasks such as dressing and showering due to pain, weakness, or de conditioning attributable to their cancer, then a referral to physical therapy may be appropriate. Patients that have specific respiratory symptoms such as shortness of breath, wheezing, or severe cough may benefit from respiratory therapy.

In addition, if the patient is having life-threatening cancer symptoms that are very difficult to control, they may be referred to a specialist team of doctors and nurses called Palliative Care. This team specializes in creating a comprehensive plan to manage pain, improve the patient's comfort and quality of life. Research studies show that early contact with a palliative care team can improve quality and duration of life. Mental health professionals such as counselors and Psychiatrists can be very helpful in treating the anxiety and depression sometimes experienced by patients. Recently there have been clinical trials demonstrating the usefulness of alternative therapies such as acupuncture and massage in treating the symptoms of the cancer itself such a pain and side effects of treatment such as nausea.

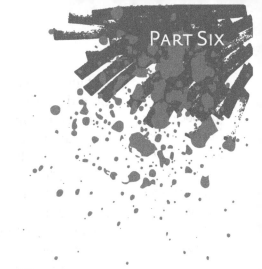

PART SIX

Focusing On Nutrition

You have been diagnosed with cancer of the lung or involving the lung(s). It's unsettling to say the least. Many patients come to me feeling initially desperate and at a loss, but it is those same patients that later say, "Hey, I'm not going to let you bully me. It's time

fig. 6.1

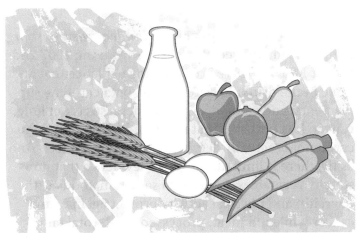

Focusing on nutrition can be the best thing that you can do for yourself during cancer therapy.

NURSE'S NOTE:

Your doctor may order a nutrition consultant for you. They can help you obtain optimal health during treatment by helping with diet, supplements, and symptom management.

to fight and I am going to do what I can to beat you or at the very least, control you so I can live my life!" Following some basic nutritional and lifestyle recommendations CAN help you in fighting lung cancer. We are going to discuss some things that can help make you feel "more in control" of what may feel like an out of control situation. What you choose to eat can have a strong impact on fighting this cancer. Your immune system is what fights off illnesses and disease. By making the best choices nutritionally, you can maximize your immune system's fighting potential. It's all about boosting your immune system, fighting inflammation, and decreasing challenges to your immune system so it can focus on the current battle at hand.

Knowledge is power. You don't know what to do if you are not informed properly, so we are here to empower you with knowledge in this fight against cancer. You will find a lot of information in this book and I want you to use it to arm yourself with knowledge. Let's get to it!

American Institute Of Cancer Research (AICR) Findings–Lung Cancer

You can visit *AICR.org* or *foodandcancerreport.org* to download, for free, the findings from the 2007 2nd Expert Report. There is convincing evidence that arsenic in the drinking water, taking beta carotene supplements, and smoking tobacco increase risk of lung cancer. It is probable that fruits and foods containing carotenoids actually decrease risk of lung cancer. And lastly, there is limited, suggestive evidence that non starchy vegetables, foods with selenium, foods with quercitin and physical activity protect against lung cancer while red meat, processed meat, total fat intake, butter, pharmacological doses of retinol (smokers only) and low body fat are associated with a higher chance of developing lung cancer.

What are you supposed to do with this information? We should be eating more foods high in selenium and quercitin, which are referred to as flavonoids, or more specifically flavonols. Selenium is found more in certain nuts and seeds and fish, while flavonols are found in vegetables and darker colored fruits. Both selenium and quercitin are naturally occurring antioxidants and are anti-inflammatory. Please see below for lists of foods containing these flavonoids.

As for the physical activity recommendations, we simply need to get moving more! Be more active and get that blood pumping! Physical activity helps directly and indirectly to decrease cancer risk. Also, it can improve mental state or mood, release negative energy and help fight inflammation. The federal guidelines for exercise are great and relatively easy to attain. It is recommended that we get physically active at least 150 minutes a week or do 75 minutes a week of vigorous exercise (if approved by your physicians). See!? Easy schmeezy! Maybe not so easy if you are undergoing treatment and are fatigued, however, we still want you to be as active as possible to help maintain muscle mass. Monitor your fatigue level and do what you can. Resistance bands are great for helping you to keep muscle tone and can be done while sitting in the comfort of your own home.

NURSE'S NOTE:

Always consult your doctor before starting a new exercise program.

Selenium Containing Foods:

Brazil nuts
Sunflower seeds
Tuna (canned light tuna in oil)
Cod (cooked)

IMMUNE BOOSTING NUTRITION

Make every bite count. Well, almost every bite. I like to follow the 80/20 rule. Eighty percent of the time you should make every bite count. Make the best choice for what you decide to fuel your body with. So often we are on the go, or in a hurry, and making unconscious decisions regarding our nutritional intake. Think about it. Is what you are eating doing anything for your body and your fight against cancer? If not, maybe you should think about making some changes in your food selections. That's not to say you can't enjoy those foods that, let's be honest, aren't good for you but they sure taste good and make you feel happy. You can. These are the foods that you have only around 20% of the time. Enjoying birthday celebrations, dessert out with girlfriends, poker night with the guys, whatever it may be, will most likely involve chips, dips and drink choices that you seldom consume. It's OK to enjoy these moments. Make a conscious effort to eat the best you can most of the time, so you can enjoy these special moments and the "not so good" nutrition choices that accompany these occasions without the guilt. It's all part of a healthy eating experience. It's all part of life, as is this current fight you've got on your hands.

Mainly, regarding your diet, the focus should lie on getting back to the basics. Having less processed foods is where it's at! When buying boxed/convenience foods, select those with fewer ingredients. Take ice cream for example. It can be a source of protein and calcium, but has high content of fat, therefore, only have it occasionally. What I want you to look at, though, is how many ingredients went into the making of it. Buy the ice cream containing only five ingredients or so. Breyers All Natural is a good example of this. I'm not saying eat ice cream all the time, but it is okay sometimes, especially if there are no chemicals/preservatives added to it. This was just an example. In general, focus on eating whole grains, dark and brightly colored fruits and vegetables, plant proteins, lean animal protein sources, fish (especially those high in Omega-3 fatty acids), and other good fats which are listed below. The idea is to balance out carbs and protein at each meal, mini meal or snack.

Whole Grains

When choosing whole grain foods, select those that have been the least processed or broken down. Some examples of whole grains include: brown rice, wild rice, whole wheat pasta, quinoa, quinoa pasta, high fiber cereals (hot or cold) containing 5 grams or more fiber per serving, and breads made from whole grain flour, having 3 grams of fiber or more per slice. Whole grain flour being the first ingredient listed. Whole grains have complex carbohydrates in them which are needed by our bodies for energy. They also have protein in them. Quinoa, for example, has 6-10 grams of protein per ½ cup. Give it a try if you haven't already.

Produce

It is recommended that 5 or more servings of fruit and vegetables be consumed each day. This is challenging for a lot of people. What I recommend is to add a fruit or vegetable to every meal, mini meal or snack eaten during the day. Try to eat small meals at 3 hour intervals. At each of these, add a serving of produce. Aim for 5 servings a day of dark or brightly colored produce.

Some of the best choices include:

- *Broccoli, cauliflower, brussels sprouts, kale and bok choy.* These are called cruciferous vegetables and they contain isothiocyanates, specifically Indole-3-Carbinol. This is a cancer fighting compound and should be consumed on a daily basis!

- *Berries* of all varieties.

- *Carrots* and orange colored produce for the carotenoids. (Carotenoid-containing foods are especially good for fighting lung cancer!)

- *Red grapes* for the resveratrol.

- *Green leafies.*

- *Tomatoes.*

This is a short list of some of the most powerful cancer fighting produce available at grocery stores. It is highly recommended you have your own garden if you can, and grow produce organically.

Plant Proteins

Foods of plant origin are high in fiber, vitamins, minerals, antioxidants, beneficial plant compounds, and pre biotic fibers to help support healthy intestinal bacteria balance. Plant based foods are the basis for an anti-inflammatory diet. Beans, legumes, lentils, nuts, seeds, soy foods—these are all sources of protein coming from a plant source. GO FOR IT! Add these to your salads, soups, chili's, or make a bean burger, etc.

Animal Proteins

Protein from animal sources is allowed also, but be sure to buy leaner cuts of meat, chicken and other poultry with no skin, and go organic when it comes to purchasing red meat and dairy products containing fat. Buy grass fed cattle because it is higher in Omega-3 fatty acids which are anti-inflammatory. Animal foods, in general, contain higher amount of Omega-6 fatty acids which are pro-inflammatory so the goal is to decrease intake of animal based foods, while we increase intake of plant based foods and fish, especially those high in Omega-3 fats. (sources listed below) *NOTE: According to the AICR (American Institute of Cancer Research 2nd Expert Report, red meat, and processed meats increase risk of lung cancer.) Why avoid processed/cured meats? Because they contain nitrates/nitrite which we know is a cancer causing preservative. This cancer causing agent is used in hams, deli meats, hot dogs, bacon and sausages.*

Select nitrate-free products such as Hormel Natural

Selections deli meat, bacon, etc and limit intake. It can be found in the deli meat section of the grocery store.

List Of Protein Foods

Beans, legumes, lentils – Typical serving size is 1/4 cup which equals 7 grams protein. Increase bean intake – try hummus spread, made from garbanzo beans (aka chickpeas).

Nuts, seeds – 1/4 cup = 7 grams protein. If nuts and seeds are not tolerated, grind nuts into a spread at your local grocery store. The nut grinders are usually found in the "Health Food" section of the grocery stores by the "All Natural" items.

Milks and spreads/nut butter made from plant foods – Almond milk, soy milk, soy yogurt, grind any nut to make a nut butter at your local grocery store.

Fish, especially wild caught salmon, tuna, halibut, mackerel and rainbow trout, for their Omega-3 fatty acid content. Omega-3s, as stated previously, are a natural anti-inflammatory and should be consumed 2-3 times per week. Other fish do not contain high levels of Omega-3s, however, are lean protein sources, with 4 ounces being a serving of fish it provides 28 grams of protein.

Eggs are a high quality protein. Each egg has about 5-7 grams of protein. Suggest having 5 eggs a week and unlimited egg whites.

Chicken and turkey, no skin, are lean protein sources. Each ounce has 7 grams protein.

LEAN cuts of red meat – Sirloin, ground sirloin for burgers vs. ground chuck, and flank steak for fajitas, for example, would be okay for consumption. Also, look for grass-fed cattle as this meat will have more Omega-3s vs. the inflammatory Omega-6s. The AICR generally recommends limiting intake of red meat, to about 3 servings per week.

Greek yogurt – has about 12-14 grams protein in it and the live cultures (probiotics) will help to normalize gut flora and promote bacteria balance in the intestines.

Low or no-fat dairy – Skim milk, 1% milk, low fat, skim mozzarella, etc. When buying a fat-containing animal product it is recommended to go organic. Look for the following statement or something similar on the label, "No hormones or antibiotics were given to this animal or used in the making of this product." Keep in mind when buying fat-containing animal foods: hormones, and toxins given to the animal are stored in the fat of the animal. The fattier the animal food, the more likely you are to consume the bad things stored in the fat of the animal. Safer to go organic when it comes to fat-containing animal products. Wise to spend your money on organic meats and dairy products.

Good Fats

Lowering dietary intake of Omega-6 fats (mostly animal foods) while raising intake of Omega-3 fats will help to shift the body into "anti-inflammatory" mode. What are good sources of Omega-3s? High Omega-3 foods include wild caught salmon, tuna, halibut, mackerel and rainbow trout. Also, foods of plant origin will have less Omega-6 fats and some Omega-3s like walnuts and flaxseed oil. Extra virgin olive oil, canola oil and coconut oil are examples of good fats as are avocados, nuts and seeds. Daily intake of a ¼-½ of an avocado is recommended.

HYDRATION

Keeping the body hydrated is so very important

NURSE'S NOTE:

Freezing your favorite foods may help you plan your meals in advance.

NURSE'S NOTE:

Remember caffeine can actually dehydrate you because it is a diuretic. You may want to cut down or eliminate caffeine completely during treatment.

every day, not just during treatment for cancer. You, in general, need 13-18 ml of non-caloric, caffeine free fluids per pound of weight each day to maintain a good hydration status. Example: 150 lbs x 13 ml/lb = 1950 ml/day which is equivalent to 8 ¼ cups per day of fluid. Monitor urine frequency, color and odor. If it looks concentrated or darker in color and has an odor, you very well may be dehydrated. On the day of chemotherapy you will receive one liter of fluid with treatment to assure you are adequately hydrated and that the chemo is flushed through your kidneys appropriately. On the other days, it is all up to you to maintain your fluid intake. If you find yourself having trouble getting enough fluid in, be sure to inform your oncologist, nurse and/or dietitian to possibly get set up for IV fluids a few days a week. Hydration is that important! It is just as important as food intake. The more vocal you are with your symptoms, the better they can be managed, so inform your health care team early and often.

BALANCE, TIMING, AND PLANNING!

Fueling your body consistently all day long, every day, will help you maintain an even keel throughout the day and avoid blood sugar peaks and valleys. By staying on an even keel all day you will provide needed support to your immune system so that it can work at its best potential. Blood sugar stabilization is key. The number one thing I hear from patients is, "I don't eat breakfast." Or, "My whole life I've never eaten breakfast." Now is the time for that to change. Try to consume calories, whether it's eating or drinking, within an hour of waking. You need to wake the body up and let it know that nutrition is on the way. If you're not doing this, it is very likely that your metabolism will slow down. Another very important thing to remember is that caffeine is an appetite suppressant. I have countless people tell me, "I just drink black coffee all morning and I'm not hungry for anything until about 4:00 in the afternoon." The reason one can go so long without having an appetite is due in part to the caffeine intake as it is suppressing the hunger cue. In actuality, you are slowing down the metabolism. What you need now is a well-oiled machine and to stay revved up to support weight maintenance as well as your immune system. We are addressing weight management and immune-boosting nutrition. To continue boosting the immune system and support your cancer fighting body, I suggest trying to eat every 3 hours, trying never to go longer than 4 hours between intake. This will help to support blood sugar stability all day long and keep you and your immune system energized. Imagine this: your body is a wood stove. You want to keep the fire burning all day long so you need logs (protein foods) and kindling (carbohydrates) every few hours. Why do this? The answer is simple. If your body doesn't have consistent source of fuel, it will think uh-oh, I don't have anything coming in, and begin to work its magic in fueling your body, slowing things down if you will and eventually pulling from energy stores in your body. You have stored energy in your muscles and when not properly nourished you may begin to breakdown muscle. A good way to gauge muscle loss is to look at your arms. Look for atrophy (shrinking muscle mass). Notice if there is any muscle or fat loss.

Of course, monitor your weight. It is okay to lose a little bit of weight but want to avoid significant weight loss. Your oncologist and care team will be following you during and after your treatment to monitor your overall health status. Significant weight loss is indicative of the inability to meet caloric needs. The registered dietitian on the team will be alerted if you should experience significant weight loss, change in nutritional status, and/or begin to be more symptomatic. A nutrition consult would be beneficial to address and possibly prevent or minimize symptoms you may encounter and provide you with ways to manage them. Managing side effects early can help to minimize the symptoms, thus minimizing the impact they may have on your overall nutritional status. It is very important to let your physician, nurse, dietitian, or any member of the health care team know of any or all symptoms you may be experiencing.

SYMPTOMS

Symptoms associated with treatment for lung cancer include: constipation (from pain meds mostly), diarrhea, decreased or no appetite, sore throat, painful swallowing, difficulty swallowing, taste changes, nausea, vomiting, shortness of breath or heavy breathing and anemia. Esophagitis may occur if radiation is part of the treatment and the location of the tumor is near the esophagus. Oftentimes, radiation therapy will be used to shrink the tumor and if the tumor is located near the esophagus, it may cause painful swelling of the esophageal area. Esophagitis is inflammation of the esophagus and can make it painful or difficult in getting foods all the way down. During radiation the body will naturally send lubrication to the site of radiation, as well as send inflammation to the radiation site. Sure the body is trying to heal this area, but it can make it difficult to swallow when there is inflammation in and around the esophagus. To manage the lubrication, which may be in the form of a sticky, thick, mucus-like phlegm, it is best to stay hydrated. Drinking water or tea constantly will provide your body with adequate fluids. This will help to thin out the secretions and make it easier to spit out if needed.

Constipation

• Drink plenty of fluids unless restricted by your doctor.

• Increase fiber intake to 25-35 grams fiber/day by eating high fiber foods such as Grape Nuts, Shredded Wheat, oatmeal, quinoa, whole grain breads and pastas, beans and lentils.

• Take acacia fiber or psyllium husk powdered supplement. Discuss with your dietitian.

• Get moving! Literally, get up and walk, stretch, be active. This will help move those bowels.

• Prunes and dried apricots tend to work well in getting the bowels moving.

• ½ cup prune juice – some like to warm it up.

• Drink fennel tea.

• Consume yogurt daily for the live cultures which will normalize gut flora. May need to take a probiotic supplement daily. First try eating yogurt 1-3 times per day.

Diarrhea

• May try L-glutamine powder. L-glutamine is an amino acid that helps repair and heal the lining of the GI tract. Take 15-30 grams/day for 2 weeks is a decent trial period.

NURSE'S NOTE:
Pain medications can be very constipating. Drink plenty of water and take a stool softener suggested by your physician to help manage this side effect.

• To replace fluids and electrolytes (sodium and potassium) lost when you have diarrhea, drink water and electrolyte replacement drinks such as Gatorade and Powerade to name a couple of examples. Pedialyte would work also. Be sure to run it by your doctor and nurse to make sure electrolyte drinks are not restricted for any reason.

• Have salty foods such as saltine crackers, broth and pretzels to replace sodium losses.

• Have foods high in potassium such as bananas, tomatoes, carrots, baked potato and plain yogurt to replace potassium losses.

• Increase soluble fiber in your diet such as applesauce, rice, bananas, and oatmeal. Acacia fiber powder is a soluble fiber that works to slowly regulate bowels.

• The only dairy foods you should have when experiencing diarrhea would be yogurt. It is recommended that yogurt be consumed 1-3 times daily to help normalize gut flora. If yogurt is not tolerated, you can take probiotic supplements in the amount of 7-15 billion live cells/day.

• Do not take vitamin C supplements when experiencing diarrhea.

Decreased or No Appetite

• Try eating small amounts of food more often throughout the day. Make every bite count by choosing high calorie and protein foods such as nuts, seeds, soybeans (edamame), maybe make a trail mix with nuts and dried fruits and even bits of dark chocolate in there. Other suggestions include: hummus spread on carrots, yogurt with low fat granola, whole grain bread with nut butter, hard boiled egg or cottage cheese and fruit.

• Take Omega-3s daily as they are anti-inflammatory and will help to counteract the inflammatory process that is making you a) not hungry, and b) when you are hungry you get full fast. Suggest 1500 mg Omega-3 fatty acids (EPA and DHA) daily.

• Eat foods high in Omega-3s such as salmon, venison, buffalo, walnuts, and use flaxseed and canola oils.

• Fruits, especially watermelon, are good to try when you are not feeling especially hungry.

• Stay hydrated with water, flavored water, 100% juice popsicles and juices.

• Smoothies, shakes and slushies are generally well-tolerated and you can pack in the calories by adding berries, fruits, carrots, milk, yogurt, protein powder, etc.

• You can drink a high calorie nutritional supplement. There are many to choose from and you can even make your own using whey or plant based protein powder. One calorie dense drink I do recommend to gain weight after a big weight loss or to prevent this from happening is Carnation VHC (Very High Calorie). This drink, unlike Ensure or Boost, is not available retail. You can ask at your cancer care facility or you can possibly contact a local home health company on your own and ask them if they carry this formula or something similar. I suggest you drink this throughout the day at a ¼ cup dose (equivalent to ¼ can), 4 times per day, refrigerating the formula in between drinks. This will equal one can total per day which is 560 calories. This can help to maintain weight, or at the very least minimize weight loss. What we don't want to happen is significant weight loss. This greatly affects your nutritional status and your fighting power.

• An appetite stimulant may be necessary for a brief amount of time. There are a couple we most commonly use, Megace or Marinol. Discuss your appetite with your doctor, nurse and dietitian so that again, we can be proactive in managing your symptoms.

• Try yoga, stretching exercises, deep breathing, Guided Imagery with a licensed counselor, talking with someone or support group, or other means of relieving stress and anxiety.

Sore throat/Painful and/or Difficulty Swallowing

• Use Magic Mouthwash. It can numb area so that you can swallow.

• Consume mostly soft foods or liquids such as puddings, mashed potatoes, eggs, pasta, oatmeal or other desired hot cereals, protein shakes/smoothies/slushies, canned peaches or pears, yogurts, and cottage cheese.

• Drink milk (skim, soy, almond, or rice milk) between meals.

• Sip soup and teas.

• Make frozen fruit sections (peaches, grapes cut in half, melons) and suck on them.

• There is something called capsaicin taffy. Capsaicin is a pain reliever and it is found in cayenne pepper. You can make it using a small amount of cayenne pepper. NEVER put cayenne pepper directly on your mouth or tongue as it is extremely spicy and hot.

Recipe is:

CAPSAICIN TAFFY

1 cup sugar
3/4 cup light corn syrup
2/3 cup water
1 tablespoon cornstarch
2 tablespoons soft margarine
1 teaspoon salt
2 teaspoons vanilla
1/2 to 1-1/2 teaspoons cayenne pepper (powdered)

Begin by using only 1/2 teaspoon of the cayenne pepper in the first recipe you make and build up to 1-1/2 teaspoons in following batches if it doesn't cause your mouth to burn. COMBINE: everything except vanilla and cayenne pepper cooking over medium heat stirring constantly, to 256 degrees Fahrenheit (use candy thermometer). Remove from heat and stir in vanilla and cayenne pepper. Once cooled enough to touch, pull taffy. Let cool on wax paper. When stiff, cut into strips, then pieces. Wrap in wax paper and store in cool, dry place.

Dry Mouth/Tender Mouth

• Sip water and teas frequently throughout the day to moisten mouth.

• Limit caffeine and alcohol intake as they tend to be a diuretic and pull fluid out of the body.

• Use a no alcohol containing mouthwash such as Biotene.

• Have water/water bottle with you at all times—take frequent sips.

• Consume moist foods such as stews, casseroles, soups, and fruits.

• Suck on ice chips, popsicles, or make slushies if cold temperature foods are desired and tolerated.

• Use broth, gravies, sauces, yogurt, silken tofu (moist and creamy), warm water, juices, milk or dairy alternatives, and coconut milk to moisten foods.

• Eat soft foods such as yogurt, all natural ice cream, oatmeal, pudding, Cream Of Wheat, Malt-O-Meal, even cooked vegetables such as cauliflower can be mashed to make "mock mashed potatoes."

• Use olive oil, canola oil, and/or coconut oil to make foods slippery and easier to swallow.

• Avoid crunchy textured foods, tough meats, and raw vegetables.

• Chew xylitol based gum. Xylitol is a sugar-free sweetener and does not promote tooth decay. This is available in most grocery stores down the "health food" or "all natural" sections of the store.

• Use a humidifier in your room at night to keep the air moist.

• Moisten lips frequently with lip balm, Aquafor, cocoa butter or olive oil.

Taste Changes

• Good oral hygiene is a must! Take good care of that mouth. A dry mouth can lead to increased bacteria growth so be sure to keep your mouth moistened and clean. If painful to brush, buy one of those sponge-ended toothbrushes and try using that for brushing.

• Mouthwash can make foods taste better. Rinse well prior to eating and see if this works for you.

• For metallic taste and dry mouth try sour food, if tolerated, such as lemon or lime in your drinking water which can work to increase saliva production, too. Eating fruits may also help to get rid of the bad taste.

• Try using plastic ware versus silverware if you have a metallic taste in your mouth.

• Cold foods such as chilled fruit, leaf salads, cold salads (egg, pasta, tuna or quinoa salads) are sometimes better tolerated if you are experiencing bitter or metallic taste changes as well as an "aftertaste."

• Try a variety of teas. Typically, mint teas do the trick to lessen bad taste changes.

• Zinc may help minimize or alleviate taste changes. Discuss Zinc supplementation with your oncologist and dietitian.

• Marinate meats, chicken and fish in a sweet marinade—sweet and sour sauce, soy/ginger/honey mixture, or raspberry vinaigrette.

Nausea and Vomiting

• Consume colorless, odorless meals, especially before

treatments. Research has shown that the meal you eat prior to treatment can make a difference in how likely you are to experience nausea and vomiting.

fig. 6.2

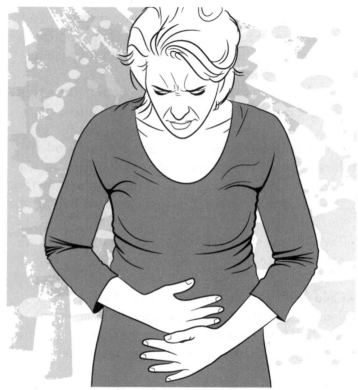

Let your providers know if you are experiencing nausea. With the many new medications available, nausea should not be a big issue for you.

• If vomiting, it is most important to focus on keeping adequately hydrated as best you can. Sip fluids every 15 minutes at least. Try clear soda, sports drinks, Pedialyte, juices, popsicles, ice chips, ginger tea or other good-sounding tea, broth, ginger ale. If you are not able to keep things down for 24 – 48 hours, please call your nurse or case manager to let them know.

• Medications are available for nausea management.

Discuss these with your oncologist and nurse.

• Eat cold foods as they are generally better tolerated and tend to not trigger vomiting.

• Stick to the old standbys: crackers, dry toast, rice, oatmeal, grits or other hot cereal.

• You can try wearing Sea Bands around your wrist. They hit a trigger point and can help lessen feeling of nausea.

NURSE'S NOTE:

If vomiting is a problem during treatment, you may need to have IV fluids a few days a week to help support you during this critical time.

Anemia

Anemia is when you do not have enough red blood cells. Red blood cells carry oxygen throughout your body and when you do not have enough you may feel tired, weak and/or short of breath. Your doctor will be monitoring your lab work to watch for anemia. There are different types of anemia such as iron deficiency anemia or it can be due to low levels of B12 and Folic acid. Sometimes anemia is caused by the cancer itself. For iron deficiency anemia, I suggest supplementing with a non-constipating iron such as ferrous bis-glycinate. Also try eating high iron foods such as meats, chicken, turkey, or fish. These are called heme sources meaning they come from the blood of the animal. There are non-heme sources like beans, lentils and green leafies. When eating these non-heme sources, have vitamin C with it to increase absorption.

Weight Loss

During treatment it will become increasingly difficult to eat. We want you to continue attempts at eating and drinking as much as possible. As mentioned before, this can be done with sips of water and

NURSE'S NOTE:

Your nurse will weigh you at least weekly during treatment. This may occur more often if weight loss is a concern.

caloric liquids such as juices, popsicles, smoothies, protein shakes or slushies, etc. To prevent weight loss and an impaired nutritional status, the use of a feeding tube is may be recommended. Try not to be alarmed. A feeding tube may be needed temporarily as a means of nourishing your body until your whole GI tract can be used. It's plain and simple, if you can't swallow your food/liquids you can't meet your nutritional needs or if part of your GI tract is not working properly nutrition support may be needed but just know all attempts to help you nourish your body the old fashioned way will be upheld. Be proactive and tell your doctor about your difficulties in eating or swallowing so that significant weight loss may be avoided or minimized. Once treatment is underway, your esophagus may become inflamed from therapy. It would be very painful to have the tube placed using an endoscope down your throat.

Tubes are placed using a variety of procedures. Some physicians only have the PEG (percutaneous endoscopic gastrostomy) placed while others have tubes placed directly into the stomach using radiologic guidance. This is an option once treatment has started, but the earlier it is placed, the less uncomfortable you will be upon placement of the tube. Be sure to discuss feeding tube possibilities and options with your doctor, registered dietitian and nurse. There are different ways to administer feedings: bolus, gravity and pump feeds. The only thing that can go in the feeding tube is liquid. There are pre-made formulas like Boost, Ensure, Fibersource, Carnation VHC, or you can make your own mixture if you like.

NURSE'S NOTE:

Ask your doctor or nurse about nutrition supplements.

SUPPLEMENTS

The AICR (American Institute of Cancer Research)

has made a recommendation to take minimal supplements while increasing nutrient density of your food intake. We do know from recent research that many of us are deficient in vitamin D. Vitamin D deficiencies are linked with cancer, MS, depression, insomnia, aches/pains, etc. Getting your vitamin D tested is highly recommended and from there it can be determined if vitamin D3 supplementation is necessary.

Fish oil, as mentioned, is often recommended because of its anti-inflammatory properties. 1500-3000 mg/day Omega-3s is recommended each day. The Omega-3s are DHA and EPA. Look for the content of these on the back of the supplement bottle. Concentrations vary greatly so be sure to take adequate amounts. If scheduled to have surgery, be sure to tell your surgeon and all physicians involved you are taking fish oil. It is recommended that fish oil be stopped prior to procedures as it thins out the blood.

A multivitamin a day is usually appropriate. Go over contents of it with your registered dietitian and/or doctor.

A fiber supplement such as acacia fiber, is beneficial if you are prone to constipation or extreme cycles of diarrhea then constipation. If you have increased fiber in your diet by incorporating whole grains, fruits and vegetables, supplementation may not be necessary.

The great debate continues on whether to take antioxidant supplementation during treatment or not. Facilities vary greatly on what is allowed or not allowed during treatment and you will need to discuss this with your oncologists. One thing I tell patients is to listen to your body. You have a mind/body connection and need to listen to it. If you feel confident that something is working for you, then do it. Don't do some supplement just because someone told you about it and it worked for them or because that is what you read on the internet. Of course you will get tons of advice at every turn, but take time to digest it all and figure out what works for you. Rather than focusing on supplementation for added nutrients, it is better to focus on maximizing your nutrient intake through food. You can go to *www.ORACvalues.com*. ORAC stands for oxygen radical absorbance capacity, which is the antioxidant power of foods. *ORACvalues.com* is a comprehensive database of foods and their antioxidant levels. Some things high in ORAC are: parsley, blueberries and cinnamon. Check out the website to see what others are high in ORAC values!

NOTE: Always discuss all meds, natural supplements, vitamins and minerals with your doctor to assure nothing is compromising your treatment.

RECOMMENDED BOOKS

Eating Well Through Cancer – distributed by Merck

The Cancer Lifeline Cookbook – by Kimberly Mathai MS, RD, with Ginny Smith

The Cancer-Fighting Kitchen and One Bite at a Time – by Rebecca Katz

In the above-mentioned books you will find whole-foods based recipes and wonderfully helpful nutrition information.

ONLINE RESOURCES

I would like to address the world of online information. You will see many things on the computer. "Googling" has become a way of life but be careful in what sites you go to. There is one theory found online that gets brought up the most. It is the theory that "sugar feeds cancer." I want you to remember one thing: anything growing inside of us will be fueled by what we are fueled by. Our main energy source is glucose. This is sugar. As stated before, follow the 80/20 rule of thumb with regards to diet and nutrition. Most definitely do not avoid fruits and whole grains in hopes of depriving your body of sugar or in hopes of starving the tumor. Keep the focus on balance of carbohydrates, proteins, and good fats. Eat whole grains, bright or dark colored produce, plant proteins, lean or lower fat animal proteins, and good fats.

RECOMMENDED WEBSITES

There are numerous websites to view. So much so it can be overwhelming. Below is a list of credible websites.

www.caring4cancer.com/go/cancer/nutrition – side effects management – written by a registered dietitian.

www.cancer.org

www.cancerrd.com

www.cancer.gov

www.nlm.nih.gov/medlineplus

www.aicr.org/site/PageServer

www.mypyramidtracker.gov/planner/

www.oralcancerfoundation.org/dental/xerostomia. htm – information on dry mouth.

www.foodnews.org – for the Dirty Dozen annual report on produce.

www.consumerlabs.com – to review your supplement. See if it passed quality testing.

www.ORACvalues.com – to review antioxidant levels of foods.

www.livestrong.org

www.asha.org/public/speech/disorders/Swallowing-Probs.htm – American Speech Language and Hearing Institute.

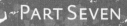

PART SEVEN

Body, Mind, Heart, Spirit

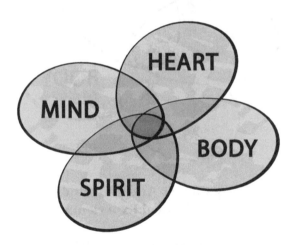

A diagnosis of lung cancer is a crisis large enough to impact your body, your mind, your heart, and your spirit. Cancer is a family disease because it affects everyone you love, and in different ways. Many people assume that a diagnosis of lung cancer is a quick death sentence, as it used to be, however today people are living longer and healthier lives than ever before. Even so, it remains a large enough crisis to change your life immediately in ways that cause you to suffer, and in other more positive ways you won't recognize until later, perhaps much later. You have a lot of work ahead as you face treatment and living with a chronic disease, as many with lung cancer must. If you think about it, curing and healing are different. The work of your physicians is to find a cure, or ways to prolong your life. You have an equally important job. Your job is to find ways and people who can help you heal the emotional and spiritual suffering generated by cancer, and to allow cancer to become your teacher. You must learn to truly live, grow, express your own needs, and have your own back.

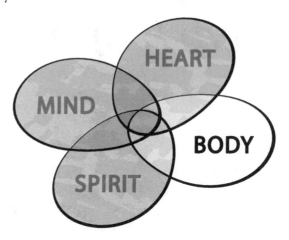

Lung Cancer And Your Body:
Your Physical Experience

"I had a pain in my breast bone. We all thought it was acid reflux. When I heard the word cancer I was stunned. It came out of nowhere. I smoked a little in college, but never seriously, and that was years ago."

"I heard the word cancer and I just wanted to stick my head in the sand. I was too exhausted to

face it. I wanted to put off treatment 'til I had more energy."

"I have a grandson! I wanted to get started with treatment immediately!"

"I smoked for years. I blamed myself for this with every breath. I hated myself. I quit smoking immediately after my diagnosis, and it was so easy. Go figure. I had tried countless times. I finally stopped hating myself when my doctor asked me this: 'Where do you want your focus to be—on blaming yourself or on healing?' I had to choose, since I couldn't focus on both. I chose healing."

"I hate my body. I hate how it feels. I hate the scars. I feel bony. I hate my hair being gone. My skin is loose. My whole body is way off. It's not me. And I have so much to do. How can I make my body DO it?"

"It takes a lot to preserve my dignity and my sense of myself now. My body is just going away. How I see myself is wearing away."

"It really bothered me that the medical staff got nicer when I mentioned that I never smoked."

He: "I don't talk about pain. I don't want to explain it all the time. I don't care about the broken dishwasher!"

She: "When he's in pain he's short tempered, grumpy and he barks at me. I need to not take it personally."

Tips For The Journey

Remember that your whole body is not sick, although it may feel like that. Aside from your lungs, how well is your body working for you now? Some people feel more hopeful when they remember that in general their body is doing well, in spite of the cancer.

Think about all the ways your body has stood by you in the past, the times you've been ill and recovered, the times your body has responded well to medical interventions, the ways your body has told you what it needs and how you have responded. You're simply doing that again, with the cancer. Your body knows how to heal.

Respect the needs of your body as you move through treatment. You will need more rest than you think. Don't push your body, which is working so hard to absorb and process different medications and procedures while maintaining normal functioning at the same time. Your body is working overtime to get you well again and to heal, which requires enormous energy. Lovingly, give it a break.

It's important to bring someone with you to doctors' appointments and treatment sessions. This needs to be someone you don't have to take care of, or entertain, or even talk to. Choose someone who can just sit and be with you, who can be another listening ear when your medical team gives you information. Research shows that people hear about 30% of the information presented to them when they are stressed, not to mention when "chemo brain" complicates memory and communication.

NURSE'S NOTE:

Some people like to journal during treatment. This helps with focus and helps them get their feelings out.

Prioritize the precious energy you have. Decide

what you want to do, then pace yourself so that you can avoid "crashing" into exhaustion and the misery that comes with that. Is completing a task most important, so that you can feel useful? Is it sharing time with a loved one that will fill your need today? Make a list of what you'd like to do. Choose. You probably can't do everything on your list, so trim in order to stay focused on what you can do, instead of what you can't. If you choose to do more than your level of energy can handle, schedule time to rest so your body can get back to healing. You'll feel more in control and content.

NURSE'S NOTE:

Talk to others who have been through the same or similar treatments. Don't worry about asking them questions.

Ask the people who love you for some ideas of things you can do that don't require physical effort. If chemo brain is holding you captive, ask for ideas for movies you might like. Funny movies are good for your immune system. War-like films might inspire the fight in you. Books with short stories or stories of how others with cancer have coped, healed or gained wisdom can help. Meet your own needs.

Allow people to help you. Be specific in your requests. People with cancer say that it's much harder to receive than to give, but remember: you are giving people a gift by receiving their help. They feel helpless, and any ways they are allowed to be helpful to you helps them, too. They are a part of your team. Relinquish thoughts that you can handle this journey alone, or that your family can manage it alone. The goal is not to endure stress, but to manage it. Receiving help is a management skill.

Perhaps most important of all, remember that you are not your disease. You are not the problem. Cancer is. You are much more than the cancer. You are a person who is loved and valued, well or sick, vital or exhausted.

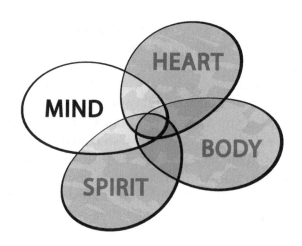

Lung Cancer And Your Mind:
Your Thoughts And Beliefs About Cancer

"My doctor said something that really helped. He said 'Don't pay any attention to statistics or anecdotal information. It's your cancer, not anybody else's."

"Cancer is not my diagnosis—it's our diagnosis. I want to protect my whole family from being scared, but it's really hard to protect them from my fears and communicate well at the same time. I keep biting my tongue."

"I'm terrified most of the time. I try not to listen to everything people say so I can stay focused on today and the next step I have to take."

"Everybody has ideas of what I should do and how I should handle this, and I don't know who to listen to."

"I'm the 'caregiver' I read about. I'm his wife. He's always asked how he's doing. People don't ask me that. Why not? I'm overwhelmed."

"I just deny that I could die. I don't even think about it. Is something wrong with me?"

"I had to change my whole perception of my cancer. I finally allowed myself to be ill. I accepted my illness, and then I could let go of so much suffering."

"I'm the key member of my medical team here. I'm the key decision maker."

"Go ahead and change doctors if you don't feel you 'click' with the doctor you have, or if you're not getting your questions answered. Do you wonder what chemo is like? Or radiation? Ask! This is your life you're fighting for!"

"The scheduler told me 'We can't get you in for two weeks' and I freaked. I wanted to yell 'Don't you understand? I'm dying of cancer here!' That was 4 years ago. I'm so thankful that urgency is gone."

"I call myself a Twinkie. I was told I had a year to live, three years ago. I've outlived my shelf life."

"I feel limited by my own thinking. I don't want to plan things. If I leave town and something goes wrong, what would I do?"

"I'm done with treatment. Am I done with cancer? How can I stay well by myself?"

"I felt the need to do the paperwork—you know, the end of life decisions—so that when I die nobody has to deal with all of that. My family was horrified that I found it comforting."

Tips For The Journey

For many there is an urge to stay silent in order to protect loved ones from powerful fears and anger, and an equally strong need to talk. Find someone you can be totally honest with, who can listen without giving advice or opinions. Allow yourself to express your fears fully so that you can let them go for now. This might be someone in your family or it might be a trusted friend. You can contact a cancer support group in your area. These are the people who really get it, since they are dealing with some of the same issues themselves. You can seek the loving ear of a spiritual advisor or a psychotherapist. Be wary of internet chat rooms and blogs. Many people become more frightened while exploring because they are exposed to other peoples' fears.

Many couples, when one partner is diagnosed with cancer, try to protect the other from their deep fears and concerns, and choose not to talk about how they are really doing. This can cause an invisible wall to descend between you, making you feel like friendly roommates instead of intimate partners. It can become harder and harder to talk honestly when this happens. Some people find themselves having the most personal conversations only with someone other than their partner, which, over time, can cause damage to the relationship. Go ahead and cry together, talk together, listen to each other's fears, and comfort each other. Get some couples counseling if you need it; this is a time of crisis. You'll feel less alone and you'll know that you're part of a team facing the cancer together. This, over time, will strengthen your relationship. Look for a caregiver support group in your area so your spouse or partner can get help with feelings of isolation, frustration, fear and guilt

NURSE'S NOTE:

Don't hesitate to let your caregivers know how you are feeling. They are there to help you.

so common to these special people whose world has turned upside down as well. The Quakers form a care committee to organize help when anyone is sick or disabled. You can do this, too.

Couples can find it helpful to talk about their relationship when one of them becomes ill. Every couple has made agreements, spoken and unspoken, about how they will be with each other. A wedding vow is such a contract. It can be helpful to clarify the unspoken assumptions you each hold about illness, what caring for each other means during illness, and what it means to give and receive support.

Be aware that some of your friends may appear to withdraw from you when they discover you have cancer. You may be thinking "When you get cancer you sure find out who your friends are". The truth is that they don't know what to say to you, or they are afraid they will cry in your presence, adding the burden of their fears or grief to your load. The longer this estrangement goes on, the guiltier they feel. Instead of feeling abandoned you could choose to initiate contact with them and let them know you miss them and would welcome their presence, in a real way, at this time.

On the other hand, there may be friends who you'd rather not be in contact with now. When you're with them you may feel their needs weighing you down, or that you need to use precious energy to attend to them. You may simply want to avoid the ubiquitous question, "How ARE you?", asked with deep concern. An option is to go online to sites such as Caring Bridge or Helping Hands, where you can enter information and updates you're comfortable sharing that others can access. This will give you more privacy and prevent you from having to answer the same questions over and over. Friends and acquaintances can send you messages this way, too.

Most people fighting cancer hear intense and heartfelt advice about which doctors to see and which alternative or complementary treatments to try. Some can be very insistent. This can be very confusing and frightening. If this kind of talk is not helpful, you can respond by saying "Thanks for your thoughts and for caring about me, but I trust the doctors I'm working with and I'm not looking for other treatments right now. I'll let you know if I change my mind." If you are interested in finding an oncology naturopath to complement your medical treatment, look online. You may be able to consult on the phone if the doctor is located at a distance.

Sometimes people say they're coping by being in denial. They are simply pacing themselves, accepting information at a speed they can tolerate as time goes by. From diagnosis through treatment, cancer is a long haul.

People with cancer are often approached by friends and coworkers who, for some reason, feel free to share the most horrifying, tragic stories of cancer suffering they know. Be prepared. You'll hear stories about relatives, friends, friends of friends, and strangers and all of the ways they suffered. Allow yourself to immediately interrupt these stories, saying something like "That story makes me feel nervous, uncomfortable, bad, or ____. Let's talk about something else."

Find ways to help yourself relax. Feeling the need to be constantly alert, ready for battle, sword in hand, is common among people facing a life-threatening disease. It can help prevent more bad news from being the kind of shock you felt at your first diagnosis. But the need to relax during your cancer journey is crucial for your healing. And the price of remaining hyper-vigilant is always feeling the threat of more cancer hanging over your head. Letting go for awhile through relaxation exercises, guided imagery, massage, meditation or prayer will help strengthen your immune system, your mood, and your ability to bring new energy to the fight. You can make this decision: "If I have to deal with cancer again, I will." Relinquish the illusion of control. Then define what truly living means for you, and step into the light.

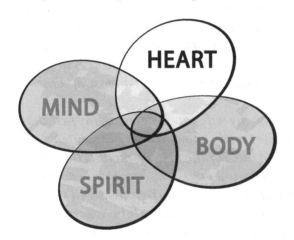

Lung Cancer And Your Heart: The Ways You Feel About Yourself, Your Life, And Cancer

"I'm so scared all the time. I've heard so many awful things about treatment. Poison, slash and burn. How will I survive this when some days all I want to do is stop?"

"I know I have to keep a positive attitude or I'll die."

"I feel so useless when I don't have any energy. I always took charge. I was the one people depended on. I just can't be that person now. I feel like such a burden on my family."

"What's the hardest loss for me, even though I've been told there's no more evidence of cancer? I'll always wonder if it will come back and kill me. I've lost forever the assumption that I'll die of old age."

"I get so scared about my medical care sometimes. If I'm unhappy with something they say or do, and I'm not nice, will they give up on me or not try so hard to save my life? I finally asked my doctor that and she was amazed. She wanted to know when I wasn't happy. So make sure you ask your questions, and insist on answers in ways you understand. It will give you a sense of control."

"When my wife was diagnosed, my first thought was 'Everybody knows it's a death sentence. She's going to die.' For the first six months there was so much fear and anger. My brain was consumed with thoughts of cancer and treatment and survival. Now, four and a half years into it, here we are, happier than we've ever been. I'm not raging at the world. Our focus is on today, on right now. We watch birds eating mountain ash berries. Did you know some birds eat them whole and others eat only the insides?"

"I'm finally mad about what cancer has done to the life I had."

"My family can get a break from the cancer by withdrawing from me for awhile. I can never get a break."

"I just can't bring myself to discipline the kids any more. I don't want to leave them with bad memories. It drives my wife crazy."

"I do the cancer stomp dance with my kids when any of us gets scared. We laugh. It helps."

"In nature, time is so different. It slows down. Don't tie time to a clock. Who knows how long any of us will live?"

"If I relax and put the fear down, the cancer will sneak up on me again. I never want to feel that shock of being diagnosed with cancer again."

"What can I count on and control? The love I give and receive. I can take this for granted when everything else is in flux."

"When I'm depressed I go somewhere else. I stop. I freeze in place and quit taking care of myself."

"I don't feel whole any more. I want the lives my friends are living."

"Losing my hair felt like one more insult. My cancer became public. I was so embarrassed. I had to become willing to just let myself be embarrassed, but in a softer way. It's not my fault this happened."

"Sex? What's that?"

"I long for the carefree days I didn't even know were carefree."

"I have regrets. I have not lived my life very fully. I've made compromises I wish I hadn't, trying to

meet other people's expectations. Cancer changed that. I'm a lot happier with myself now."

"I want to leave a legacy of good work. I may need to leave my work unfinished, unresolved. That breaks my heart."

"When I was first diagnosed I was so stressed I felt close to suicide. I didn't want to hurt anybody, but I just wanted to feel some peace. Then, after a couple of treatments I thought 'OK, I can do this.' I felt much more relaxed. Now, after several years, I don't think about cancer. I think instead about each day. I focus on one day, one symptom at a time."

"I'm learning to check inside and ask myself 'What is the truth here and what is the fear?' I try to separate them now."

"Cancer is like the holocaust, or the tsunami. God wasn't mad at all those people who died."

"It's not about dying somewhere down the road. It's about loving her now. Worrying about her dying is wasting precious time. To people just hearing they have lung cancer, or any cancer, I'd say 'You will get to a place where you know this and are more at peace. I promise."

Tips For The Journey

It will help if you think back on the hardest times you have already survived in your life. How did you make it through? What coping skills did you depend on? Did you need to talk, or withdraw for awhile? Did you allow yourself to feel sad, or angry? Did gathering information help? Did you need to turn the whole thing over to the "professionals" to "fix" so that you could relax? Did you have ways to distract yourself when you needed that? Did you pray? Did you allow people who loved you to help you? How? What worked back then? Tell a trusted friend the stories of how life has taught you these skills.

NURSE'S NOTE:

Stay in contact with people you love. Keep your mind active.

Think about the strengths of character you bring to this challenge. Recognize your wisdom, your inner power, your determination. What qualities did you bring to the critical times you've already survived in your life? If you're not sure, ask people who love you. They often see us more clearly than we see ourselves, especially when we are anxious. And, again, tell the stories of how life taught you to find these strengths within yourself.

There is a difference between grief and depression. When we grieve we know exactly why we feel so low. When we are depressed we often live in a cloud of unease and sadness without really knowing why. Sometimes people feel both. Things that used to bring you pleasure, or even deep joy, may feel empty now. Grieve through the losses that treatment has forced upon you. Meetings with a counselor can help you figure out where you are stuck, ways that might help you feel more centered and peaceful, and whether an anti-depressant would help for the time being.

Conflict often happens in families when differing ways of coping with the cancer collide. It is important to allow people to cope in their own ways. For example, one person may be devastated by fears that you will die. Another may be totally focused on what you need to do to complete treatment. Or, one person, in order to relax, may need to hear every update, attend all of your doctors' appointments and treatment sessions. For others, this might cause unbearable stress. The statements to avoid among family members are: "You shouldn't feel that way" and "If you love ___ (the person with cancer) enough you'd ___".

Remember this: you are not the burden weighing on the people who love you. The cancer is burdening all of you. For every family, when cancer is diagnosed, the fear of death is real, painful, and lasting. This is called anticipatory grief and it happens when any loved one's life is threatened, whether they die from the disease or not. That is part of the burden cancer places on all of you. Ask someone close to you to remind you of this, that you are not the burden, when you forget it. Most people do.

Children around the age of five (and older) always wonder if their parent is going to die from the cancer. Many of them will come right out and ask, while others hold this secret dread deep inside, causing physical symptoms or fears of going to school and leaving you alone at home. Children also wonder if they caused your cancer. This is what your children need from you: to know that they are loved and will be cared for by someone they trust during those times when you can't. They need to continue their normal routines such as music lessons and sports practices and games. The family rules, like bedtimes, time spent on computer games, etc., need to be maintained as closely as possible. Your children need to hear these promises from you: "I promise that the cancer is not your fault. I promise that I will tell you if I'm going to die from the cancer. Dying is not something the doctors are worried about at all now. So you don't need to worry about it. I want you to promise in exchange that you will come and talk with me when you are scared about this or anything else. I want to hear from you about anything else you want to talk to me about, too."

Learn to receive. Many people find this to be embarrassing, and question whether they deserve what their loved ones want to give. How can we learn to receive? Sometimes cancer forces the issue. For example, when you just cannot do the things necessary for your own well being, you have to ask for help. Other times, you can ease into it, intentionally receiving a bit, then more (like having a friend take your children to soccer practices). Ask yourself: would your loved ones deserve to receive help and care from you, were your circumstances reversed? Then why not you? Consider this: how would you feel if they refused your offer of help? Cancer, thankfully, has a way of severely disrupting the perfectionist standards many of us learned in childhood.

Depend on your loved ones. They want you to. Let them know what you'd like them to do for you. You could even ask them to do something you would do if you could for someone else. One woman had her sister tell their mother about the recurrence so that she would not have to see the look on her mother's face. That way she didn't have to bear the full load of disclosing the bad news. Avoid expressing your gratitude constantly, in a guilty way. Let yourself receive. One heartfelt thank you is enough.

One of the ways people stay balanced while living with cancer is to imagine their hands held open before them, one holding the reality "I might live. I just might live." The other hand holds the reality "This cancer might take my life long before I ever thought I'd die." Those who grasp only the possibility of living can become very anxious, for the opposite reality is also possible. Those who grasp only the possibility of dying sooner than they hoped can become stuck in depression. Hold both possibilities, lightly if you can, and remember: the weights in your hands will fluctuate, back and forth. The days you feel dispirited and down won't last. The days you feel filled with hope and confident you'll do well won't either. Remember the cancer motto: "Right now I'm OK. If that changes I'll deal with it, because that's what I do."

Feeling embarrassed about hair loss or looking as exhausted as you feel can be very hard. When friends ask if there is something they can do for you, you might suggest they take you to buy a beautiful scarf, or spend some time with a make-up specialist. You could suggest a scarf party be held for you. Have the organizer suggest people buy only soft, cotton scarves for you, since they won't slip on your head when your hair is gone. You may feel more at peace with your appearance if you surrender to it and find ways to kindly see yourself through the long walk of hair re-growth and energy renewal, replacing critical self-talk with kindness and acceptance, in soft and loving tones.

Sexuality. So many people struggling with side effects from treatment are upset about the sudden and what feels like permanent, irrevocable disappearance of their sexual feelings. Feelings of guilt can exist for both partners, one for not wanting to make love, the other for wanting to. Talk together about ways that are comfortable and meaningful to physically express your love. The spontaneity of love-making can feel lost, but remember when you first began your sexual relationship? For many, there was nothing spontaneous about it. You spent time and effort preparing, lighting candles, choosing what to wear, selecting special music. When cancer treatment is done, your sexual feelings may well return, and for many couples, getting through such a crisis together has strengthened their relationship so that love making becomes an even deeper, more loving experience than it was before.

Beware of something that might be called "the positive trap". No doubt you have heard the well-meaning advice, "Be positive!", many times, in many ways. People with cancer fear that if they are not thinking positively they will not get well, and might even die. But the opposite is true. Research shows that holding in the "negative" feelings such as anxiety, anger or sadness can be harmful to immune function in an indirect way. Expression of emotions—all of them—is an important part of staying healthy throughout the cancer journey. It is important to know someone who can listen to all of your emotions, hopeful and not, without imparting judgment or fear. By expressing them, you can let the scary feelings go and learn to take one day, or even one moment, at a time. Remember this cancer motto: "In this moment I am OK. If that changes I'll deal with it, because that's what I do." Tape this to a place where you will see it every day. Remember it. It's true.

People express emotions in a variety of ways. You may need to cry or you may feel relieved simply to acknowledge or describe your feelings of sadness. Men and women are often different in this way. No one way is better than another.

There are other benefits of expressing your fears, anger and sadness with someone you trust. When you do, hope that was hidden under those feelings bubbles up to the surface of your awareness. Expressing fears frees the hope to rise.

Sometimes people with cancer feel their hopes have died. Hopes that cannot be realized die, but new hopes always wait in the wings for us to discover them. What are you hoping for today? Make a list of your hopes, the ones that will make today better, and the big ones you hope to be fulfilled down the road. Review your list frequently, revise it, and share it with someone you're close to. This can lighten your spirit, and help define what you choose to do with the energy you have to use today.

When you become most discouraged, call a meeting with your closest friends and ask them to tell you why they want you to live. Allow their words to sink into you, encourage you, give you comfort, and inspire you.

Consider joining a cancer support group. Although you are unique in your experience of cancer, the other group members are the only people who can come close to really understanding how you feel.

If you're not drawn to a support group, you can ask one of your medical providers, like your oncologist, a nurse, or the oncology counselor to contact another person with lung cancer and ask if he or she would be willing to contact you. Many people going through or finishing treatment themselves volunteer to call others who could use a listening ear. These relationships can become special and powerful sources of support, encouragement, and understanding.

Consider asking your care team for a referral to an oncology family therapist or counselor who can see you individually or include your family and other loved ones. Such a person can explore ways of coping that will work for you and help you all manage the many, sometimes conflicting ways people cope with their fear of losing someone they love and depend upon.

An experience of cancer changes people and the lives they are living, as we have seen. When it comes to managing your life after cancer, when treatment is completed, it can help to redefine your whole life, as daunting as that sounds. Take adequate time to think, write, and talk about what your "new normal" life looks like, exploring this idea as it relates to your body (what you can do to keep it well), your mind (how you are thinking differently about your life, what thoughts sustain you and nourish you now), your heart (how you take care of yourself emotionally when you fear a recurrence, and how you let others love you in new ways now), and your spirit (how you think and feel differently about God and spirituality in your life after treatment is done). A "new normal" life is made up of what has changed because of the cancer, and includes what you have lost as a result of cancer, what you have gained as a result of cancer, what you are choosing to let go of as a result of cancer, and what you are choosing to let in now, as a result of cancer.

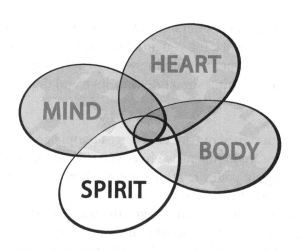

Lung Cancer And Your Spirit: The Ways You Think And Feel About God And Your Spirituality

"Lung cancer blew my spirit open. It made me embrace what I already knew, but be it and think it more, thankfully. I know I'm not alone, ever."

"I've never been religious or spiritual. It was never part of my upbringing. But I don't know where to turn to inside myself now."

"Before, I was angry at God for my early life. I stopped being angry at God when I got cancer."

"I get restless in church for the first time in my life. I used to love it. It feels meaningless to me now, and I don't know why. That scares me. I've lost God."

"My mind likes to take control, and then connection to my spirit feels lost. Cancer has forced me inside, into this moment. Then I can find myself again."

"I'm still looking for spiritual tools. I want a con-

nection with God on a more consistent basis, every day. No matter what I'm facing I want to have a sense of peace about it. I pray for peace."

"I envy my friends who have what they call 'faith'. When there is nowhere to look, where do I look?"

"Security is knowing that we have none, except for God."

"I learned how to fight, and hang on, and find solutions along the way. But now I'm told it's time to call Hospice. How can I let go of all I've learned and let myself die?"

"If I don't stop trying to control what I can't control–the cancer–and resent it, and be angry at it, I'll never heal into the kind of person I want to become. I want something good to come out of this whether I make it out alive or not."

"I'm trying to forgive myself for wasting the gifts I was given in this life. I could have done more, made more of an impact."

"I learned very well to get through years of cancer by living one day at a time, looking only at the small picture of what was immediately demanded of me. Now it seems I have to say goodbye and look at the big picture again. Where am I going? That is hard to do."

"My wife and I look at the circle of life. Dying goes on every minute of every day, everywhere. It's normal and natural. It's easy to see that in nature. That comforts me."

Tips For The Journey

In our lives, we all face three sets of lessons that teach us wisdom: the lessons of the dark (learning to let go of thoughts and beliefs that no longer fit or are hurtful to ourselves, and learning to feel whole in solitude), lessons of light (learning to let love in and hold on to it, walking through the fire that burns away our defenses, allowing for the depth and joy of emotional and spiritual intimacy) and lessons of the gray (learning to simply wait when we have already leaped into mid-air, relinquishing what no longer works well, but haven't yet landed at the next level of understanding or peace. This is practicing spiritual patience, and it's one of the most difficult tasks of all.)

It is common for people who are facing a trauma or crisis with no quick resolution to feel lost in the wilderness of their experience, beyond the reach of God. This can happen even as belief in God and in the power of God's love remain clear and strong. The feelings of loss and the impulse to justify the loss with thoughts of cancer as punishment can be devastating. What may be true instead is that when we fall off a cliff, so to speak, and are in a deeper, darker place than we've ever known, we need to do the important work of allowing God to find us. God seeks us, just as we seek God. Again, this can be a time of waiting, and the work is learning spiritual patience.

Many people do not consider themselves religious, or even spiritual. If this is true for you, it might help to define, clarify and focus on which values mean the most to you, and the beliefs that have sustained you throughout your life. How have you used these values to guide your choices during difficult experiences in the past? What have you learned about yourself having survived past crises? What gives your life meaning now? Where do you find hope now?

If the idea of faith is new and appealing, talk with people whose faith you admire, whose faith guides the choices they make. Let them be the first of many teachers.

When you feel most afraid or disheartened, what do you need to remember? What spiritual beliefs can you lean into now? Close your eyes and softly allow them to hold you, surround you, and fill you with peace. Allow all of the stress and anxiety to flow through you, going on its way without you. Become the boulder in the river of fear.

What are you praying for? Many people find their prayers changing as they move through the experience of cancer. From prayers of pleading and longing, based upon fears, they find themselves simply asking for strength to move to the next step, trust to help manage fear, or the wisdom to allow the journey to take the path it needs to take, and the time it requires. Some simply ask for help.

Do you pray for yourself? Many people do not, and consider doing so to be selfish. Yet, when it comes to our spiritual health, we need to ask for what we want, and open to the answers as they come. You may become more comfortable seeking on your own behalf if you allow yourself to ask for qualities you need to be able to grow spiritually through the experience of cancer. For example: "Please help me to always feel Your presence in my heart...teach me to feel the peace I know is there, waiting behind my fears...fill me with trust in those who are working to make me better...give me patience and tolerance to bear this vulnerability...". Then you need to become aware of these qualities coming alive inside you. Asking is only half of the process.

Some say that prayer is speaking with God, while meditation is listening to God. You might decide to meditate. Mindfulness Meditation, practiced daily for 8 weeks, has been shown on MRIs to increase the amount of brain matter in the part of the brain where we manage fears. Such a practice trains our brains to let go of frightening thoughts, so they are no longer as capable of "kidnapping" our minds. Meditation teaches us to bring our attention to the present moment, when our lives can feel safe. It is fore thoughts of loss that cause us to worry.

When it comes time to die, we prepare ourselves. Hospice workers consistently hear patients say things that reflect a growing peace about letting go of this precious life, beloved families and loved ones, and work left unfinished. We somehow come to understand, when it is time to move on, that we have left enough of a legacy behind, that the energy of our passion for life is palpable and available for those we are leaving, and it is enough. How can this happen? Perhaps it is because we finally learn that being, when we can no longer do, illuminates an enhancement of our life energy, not a diminishment.

In Summary...

Learning to live and thrive with lung cancer requires that you focus on all the parts of your life—how you act, how you think, how you feel, and how you let yourself be loved—so that you can flow through this life altering experience, and arrive at a better place afterward, knowing your ability to heal and your own wholeness more deeply than you ever knew them before. For your body: rest, exercise, massage (with an oncology trained massage therapist), guided imagery (which is a journey inside your mind which can positively impact your body) yoga, acupuncture, relaxing breathing techniques and other complementary services can help. For your mind: cognitive behavioral therapy, family therapy, and seeking the guidance of those who have walked this path before you can diminish much of the stress. For your heart: emotional support, learning to cast a loving eye on yourself, family therapy, and seeking the wisdom of the wisest people you know, and the guidance of those who have been there, can help create your new path. For your spirit: prayer, consultations with spiritual teachers, developing a meditation practice, and silent retreats may illuminate the way ahead.

Because of the cancer, you and the people you love have been forced to consider the possibility of your death earlier than any of you would have thought necessary. As difficult and frightening as this is, it is also a gift. As you consider coming to terms with dying, you gain the wisdom of this journey earlier, and it can have an intentional positive impact on your own future and on the future of everyone who loves you. However you choose to move forward, encouraging yourself to fight the cancer and not yourself, and allowing yourself to receive in all of the ways mentioned above, will make a difference in both the quality of your journey now, and the feelings of peace which await.

Resources

Kitchen Table Wisdom by Rachel Naomi Remen MD

The Anxiety and Phobia Workbook by Edmund Bourne PhD

The Wisdom of No Escape by Pema Chodron

Comfortable With Uncertainty by Pema Chodron

The Places That Scare You by Pema Chodron

Final Gifts by Maggie Callanan

Healthjourneys.com for guided imagery CDs, using your mind to impact your body

American Cancer Society

Inspire.com

CaringBridge.com

HelpingHands.com

pandora.com (radio): Calm Meditation music

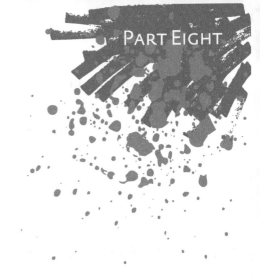

PART EIGHT

Your Cancer Journal

YOUR WORKBOOK TO
COLLECT INFORMATION

Date of my diagnosis with cancer? _____

What type of cancer do I have? _____

Where did it start? _____

Has it spread to any other areas? _____

Where has it spread? _____

What is my cancer stage? _____

T_____N_____M_____

What are my current medications and doses?

1. _____

2. _____

3. _____

4. _____

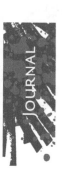

I am allergic to these medications:

1. _____

2. _____

3. _____

What treatment have my health care providers recommended?

Surgery? _____

Radiation? _____
(Type and for how long)

Chemotherapy? _____
(Type and for how long)

Who are the care providers on my team? (Phone #)

1. _____

2. _____

3. _____

4. _____

5. _____

Record questions to be asked:

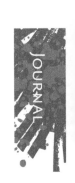

Notes and drawings:

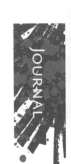

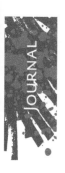

Record dates and times of new symptoms for your records:

New Symptoms	Date And Time	Severity (1-10)

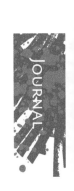

JOURNAL

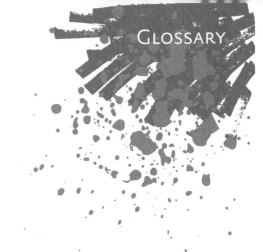

Common Cancer Terms

Adenocarcinoma: Cancer that originates from the glandular tissue of the body.

Adjuvant therapy: Treatment used in addition to the main form of therapy. It usually refers to treatment utilized after surgery. As an example, chemotherapy or radiation may be given after surgery to increase the chance of cure.

Angiogenesis: The process of forming new blood vessels. Some cancer therapies work by blocking angiogenesis, and this blocks nutrients from reaching cancer cells.

Antigen: A substance that triggers an immune response by the body. This immune response involves the body making antibodies.

Benign tumor: An abnormal growth that is not cancer and does not spread to other areas of the body.

Biopsy: The removal of a sample of tissue to detect whether cancer is present.

Brachytherapy: Internal radiation treatment given by placing radioactive seeds or pellets directly in the tumor or next to it.

Cancer: The process of cells growing out of control due to mutations in DNA.

Carcinoma: A malignant tumor (cancer) that starts in the lining layer of organs. The most frequent types are lung, breast, colon, and prostate.

Chemotherapy: Medicine usually given by an IV or in pill form to stop cancer cells from dividing and spreading.

Clinical Trials: Research studies that allow testing of new treatments or drugs and compare the outcomes to standard treatments. Before the new treatment is studied on patients, it is studied in the laboratory. The human studies are called clinical trials.

Computerized Axial Tomography: Otherwise known as a CT scan. This is a picture taken to evaluate the anatomy of the body in three dimensions.

Cytokine: A product of the immune system that may stimulate immunity and cause shrinkage of some cancers.

Deoxyribonucleic Acid: Otherwise known as DNA. The genetic blueprint found in the nucleus of the cell. The DNA holds information on cell growth, division, and function.

Enzyme: A protein that increases the rate of chemical reactions in living cells.

Excision: Surgical removal of a tumor.

Feeding tube: A flexible tube placed in the stomach through which nutrition can be given.

Gastro esophageal Reflux Disease (GERD): A condition in which stomach acid moves up into the esophagus and causes a burning sensation.

Genetic Testing: Tests performed to determine whether someone has certain genes which increase cancer risk.

Grade: A measurement of how abnormal a cell looks under a microscope. Cancers with more abnormal appearing cells (higher grade tumors) have the tendency to be faster growing and have a worse prognosis.

Hereditary Cancer Syndrome: Conditions that are associated with cancer development and can occur in family members because of a mutated gene.

Histology: A description of the cancer cells which can distinguish what part of the body the cells originated from.

Image-Guided Radiation Therapy: Also called IGRT. The process of obtaining frequent images during radiation therapy. These are used to position the radiation accurately.

Immunotherapy: Treatments that promote or support the body's immune system response to a disease such as cancer.

Intensity Modulated Radiation Therapy: Also known as IMRT. A complex type of radiation therapy where many beams are used. It spares surrounding normal tissues and treats the cancer with more precision.

Leukemia: Cancer of the blood or blood-forming organs. People with leukemia often have a noticeable increase in white blood cells (leukocytes).

Localized cancer: Cancer that has not spread to another part of the body.

Lymph nodes: Bean shaped structures that are the "filter" of the body. The fluid that passes through them is called lymph fluid and filters unwanted materials like cancer cells, bacteria, and viruses.

Malignant: A tumor that is cancer.

Mediastinum: The lymph node bearing areas in the center of the chest between the lungs and above the heart.

Metastasis: The spread of cancer cells to other parts of the body such as the lungs or bones.

Monoclonal Antibodies: Antibodies made in the lab to work as homing devices for cancer cells.

Mutation: A change in the DNA of a cell. Cancer is caused by mutations in the cell which lead to abnormal growth and function of the cell.

Neoadjuvant therapy: Systemic and/or radiation treatment given before surgery to shrink a tumor.

Osteoradionecrosis (Osteonecrosis): Damage to bone resulting from radiation doses.

Palliative treatment: Treatment that relieves symptoms, such as pain, but is not expected to cure the disease. Its main purpose is to improve the patient's quality of life.

Pathologist: A doctor trained to recognize tumor cells as benign or cancerous.

Positron Emission Tomography: Also known as a PET scan. This test is used to look at cell metabolism to recognize areas in the body where the cancer may be hiding.

Radiation therapy: Invisible high energy beams that can shrink or kill cancer cells.

Resection: Surgical removal of a tumor.

Recurrence: When cancer comes back after treatment.

Remission: Partial or complete disappearance of the signs and symptoms of cancer. This is not necessarily a cure.

Risk factors: Environmental and genetic factors that increase our chance of getting cancer.

Side effects: Unwanted effects of treatment such as hair loss, burns or rash on the skin, sore throat, etc.

Simulation: Mapping session where radiation is planned. If the doctor will be using a mask for your treatment, this is the time it will be custom fit for your face.

Staging: Tests that help to determine if the cancer has spread to lymph nodes or other organs.

Standard Therapy: The most commonly used and widely accepted form of treatment that has been tested and proven.

Targeted Therapy: Modern cancer treatments that attack the part of cancer cells that make them different from normal cells. Targeted agents tend to have different side effects than conventional chemotherapy drugs.

Tumor: A new growth of tissue which forms a lump on or inside the body that may or may not be cancerous.

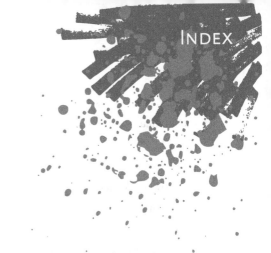

About The Authors

Barbara Gitlitz, MD: After graduating with an MD degree from the State University of New York Stony Brook, Dr. Gitlitz moved out west to California. After completing a Fellowship in Hematology Oncology and Translational Investigation at UCLA, she stayed on as an Assistant Professor. Much of her early clinical-translational work involved cancer immunotherapy including one of the first trials of a Dendritic Cell Vaccine for patients with kidney cancer. She then joined the Keck School of Medicine at USC as an Associate Professor to spearhead the USC oncology effort in lung cancer and head and neck cancer. Her most rewarding part of working at USC is being a member of multidisciplinary treatment teams; where medical oncologists, surgeons, radiation oncologists and other specialists can collaborate together on the best, individualized treatment plan for a patient.

Her dedicated, compassionate clinical care has been noticed by the community as she has been consistently nominated to the list of Los Angeles Magazine Superdoctors, Pasadena Magazine Top Doctors, and US News Top Doctors. She has received research grants from the American Cancer Society, the National Institute of Health and STOP cancer. Currently she is a member of the Stand Up 2 Cancer Epigenetics Dream Team where she will bring novel trials to treat lung cancer with combinations of immunotherapy and therapy to awaken important genes that are "turned off" by growing cancers. Dr. Gitlitz has a passion for working with scientists seeking ways to personalize therapy and bring novel drugs (clinical trials) to treat her patients. She believes that each person's cancer may have unique molecular/genomic features to help guide the best treatment plan.

125

Daniel S. Oh, MD: Daniel is an Assistant Professor of Surgery in the Division of Thoracic Surgery at the Keck School of Medicine, University of Southern California in Los Angeles. He is an attending surgeon at the Keck Medical Center of USC with a focus in thoracic surgical oncology. He has a specific interest in applying minimally invasive and robotic techniques in the care of his patients. He obtained his B.A. in English with High Honors at Wesleyan University in Middletown, Connecticut. He then obtained his M.D. at the Stritch School of Medicine of Loyola University of Chicago, where he was elected to the Alpha Omega Alpha medical honor society. He trained in general surgery at the University of Southern California and in thoracic surgery at the Brigham and Women's Hospital/Harvard Medical School.

Amol Rao, MD: Amol completed his MD degree from the St. George's School of Medicine and subsequently completed his Internal Medicine training at the SUNY Health Science Center at Brooklyn. He then spent time at the University of California, Los Angeles researching novel immune modulating therapies in melanoma with several of the projects leading to recently FDA approved drugs. He is currently Chief Fellow while completing his Fellowship in Hematology and Oncology at the Keck School of Medicine of USC and the LA County-USC Medical Center.

Stephen V. Liu, MD: Stephen is currently an Assistant Professor of Medicine in the Division of Medical Oncology at the University of Southern California Norris Comprehensive Cancer Center. Dr.. Liu graduated cum laude from Johns Hopkins University and received his medical degree from the University of Maryland. He then completed his internal medicine training at the University of Pennsylvania before receiving his fellowship training in hematology and oncology at the University of Southern California. He then joined the faculty at USC where he maintains a busy clinical practice.

Dr.. Liu specializes in lung cancer and cancers of the head and neck. His research focuses on understanding the molecular mechanisms of cancer progression and resistance to therapy. He has a particular interest in the development of personalized treatment strategies for all types of cancer. Dr.. Liu serves as the principal investigator on several clinical trials evaluating promising new drugs. He has authored a large number of peer-reviewed articles, book chapters and abstracts in several areas of research.

Dr.. Liu is originally from Pittsburgh, PA but currently resides in Los Angeles, CA with his wife.

O. Kenneth Macdonald, MD: Kenneth is a board-certified Radiation Oncologist who practices full-time in Kansas City, KS as a partner in Therapeutic Radiologists, Inc. PA. He previously was a Consultant at Mayo Clinic, Rochester,

MN, where he assisted in developing brachytherapy and stereotactic radiation techniques. He currently serves as Medical Director in the department of radiation oncology at Providence Medical Center.

Dr.. Macdonald has developed and implemented clinical trials in prostate, gynecologic and lung cancers. He an author in over 30 peer-reviewed articles and has presented his findings both nationally and internationally. His clinical interests include Lung Cancer and stereotactic radiotherapy applications.

Wayne T. Lamoreaux, MD: Dr.. Lamoreaux, was born in Southern California and spent his formative years in Arizona. After graduating magna cum laude from Utah State University in 1996, he completed medical school at the University of Utah in 2000, and then fulfilled a one year internship in Spokane Washington. In 2005, he finished a four year Radiation Oncology Residency at Washington University in St. Louis, where he served as Chief Resident, and was awarded the RSNA Roentgen Resident/Fellow Research Award. He is a board-certified Radiation Oncologist and current President of Cancer Care Northwest, a regionally comprehensive, multi-specialty oncology physician group located in Spokane, Washington. They run four integrated cancer centers and seven outreach clinics throughout the Inland Northwest.

Throughout his career, he has maintained leadership and research interests aimed at improving the treatment and the outcome of patients with cancer. He has coauthored multiple scientific articles and book chapters and presented his work at national and international meetings. He is married with four children, is fluent in Spanish, and enjoys soccer, snow skiing and water sports.

Robert K. Fairbanks, MD: Dr.. Fairbanks is the son of an Educator/Sculptor from Southeastern Arizona. His undergraduate studies were in cell biology at Arizona State University. During his undergraduate studies he was awarded two patents for work in semiconductor research. From 1988 to 1992 he attended Tulane University School of Medicine in New Orleans during which time he was awarded research grants from the American Heart and the American Diabetes Associations. During Medical School he completed a two month Lymphoma Research assignment at the Mayo Clinic. After Graduation from medical school, he served as Chief Resident and completed his internship in the transitional residency program at Tulane Medical Center. His Radiation Oncology residency training was completed at Johns Hopkins Hospital in Baltimore where he again served a year as Chief Resident. He then took a position as an Associate Professor of Radiation Oncology with Texas A&M Medical School. Subsequently he practiced Radiation Oncology in Everett, WA and now is with Cancer Care Northwest a multi-disciplinary Cancer Clinic in Spokane, WA.

He is a Board Certified in Therapeutic Radiology/Radiation Oncology. He has interest in clinical research, and has coauthored multiple scientific articles. He has special interest in intracranial and body radiosurgery & intraoperative radiotherapy/brachytherapy. He maintains outside interest in art, travel and scuba diving.

Jason A. Call, MD: Dr.. Call attended Brigham Young University where he graduated cum laude in 2003 with a double major in Zoology and Russian. He received an M.D. in 2007 from the Medical College of Wisconsin. He participated in a summer research fellowship in the Department of Radiation Oncology during his medical school education. After completing an internship year at Aurora St. Luke's Medical Center, he went on to receive four more years of training in Radiation Oncology at the Mayo Clinic in Rochester, MN. He also has special training in Gynecologic Brachytherapy that was completed at the American Brachytherapy Society School of GYN Brachytherapy in Chicago, IL.

Throughout his career Dr.. Call has been active in clinical oncology research. He has presented his research at national and international oncology meetings, published scientific papers in peer reviewed journals, and has published chapters for Oncology textbooks. He joined Cancer Care Northwest as a Radiation Oncologist in 2012.

Heather Gabbert, MS, RD, LD, CD: Heather attended Southern Illinois University at Carbondale and graduated with her Master's Degree in Dietetics in 1995. She has been a Registered Dietitian (RD) for 17 years and has lived in different areas of the country throughout the years, in each place, gaining valuable experience in the field of dietetics. She has worked with cancer patients since 1998 when she began working at Cancer Treatment Centers of America. She continued to work intermittently for CTCA throughout the many years she has been a practitioner. Heather moved to Spokane, Washington, from Chicago, Illinois, in 2007 where she works as an RD for Cancer Care Northwest and a home health company. Professionally, Heather's passion lies in working with cancer patients and promoting wellness and disease prevention for all.

Heather is a member of Academy of Nutrition and Dietetics (AND), Washington State Academy of Nutrition and Dietetics (WSAND), and Greater Spokane Dietetics Association (GSDA). She served for two years as Media Representative and board member for WSAND and GSDA. Heather has authored a book, been a contributing writer, written articles and was a blogger for StepUpSpokane, highlighting nutrition and wellness. She is a member of AND's DPG groups: Oncology, Business Communications and Entrepreneurs, Dietitians in Integrative Medicine, and Sports, Cardio and Wellness Nutrition (SCAN) group.

Heather most enjoys time spent with her two children. She also enjoys life as a Zumba instructor, exerciser and most memorable activities are her first half marathon and participating in an adventure race, which involved trail-running, biking and kayaking.

Tess Taft, MSW, LICSW: Tess is an oncology stress management specialist and family therapist who has served cancer patients and their loved ones in hospitals, cancer clinics, homes, nursing homes, hospices and private practice settings for 34 years. She received a Masters Degree in Social Work from The University of Washington in 1979 and completed a Marriage and Family Therapy training program in 1981. In 1990 she became a certified specialist in Interactive Guided Imagery for Medical Clinicians in order to teach clients this unique and powerful tool to help with symptom and stress management, and to explore and deepen hope and faith. She has taught a Palliative Care certification program for graduate social work students at Eastern Washington University since 2007, which includes 3 classes: Family Systems and Illness, Death and Dying, and Alternatives in Healing. Tess has provided trainings nationally, as well as clinical supervision for many therapists over the years. She is committed to serving people whose life-threatening diagnosis, or that of a love, has propelled them on a journey inside themselves to find emotional and spiritual healing and peace.

Kathy Beach, RN: Kathy graduated with her RN degree in 1993. She decided to get a degree in nursing after her mother was diagnosed with breast cancer. She spent sixteen years in hospital nursing where she worked on a wide range of units from Medical Oncology to Outpatient Surgery. For the past 4 years, she has focused her energy in oncology and radiation oncology with Cancer Care Northwest in Spokane, WA. She loves her work and finds the patients she cares for and their families to be extremely inspiring.

Christopher M. Lee, MD: Dr.. Lee is a practicing Radiation Oncologist and is the Director of Research for Cancer Care Northwest and The Gamma Knife of Spokane (Spokane, WA). Dr.. Lee graduated cum laude in Biochemistry from Brigham Young University in 1997 which included a summer research fellowship at Harvard University and Brigham and Women's Hospital. He subsequently attended Saint Louis University School of Medicine where he received his M.D. with Distinction in Research degree. He completed four additional years of specialty training in Radiation Oncology at the Huntsman Cancer Hospital and University of Utah Medical Center during which he was given multiple national awards. Dr. Lee has actively pursued both basic science and clinical research throughout his career. He continues to be a proliferative author of scientific papers and regularly gives presentations on radiotherapy technique and the use of targeted radiation in the care of patients with head and neck (throat), brain, breast, gynecologic, and prostate malignancies.

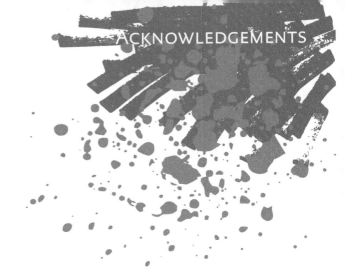
This patient handbook is the lung cancer volume of the "Living And Thriving With..." series.

We greatly appreciate the educational grant by

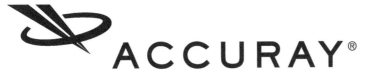

ACCURAY®

which largely funded the development of this patient centered guidebook.

CPSIA information can be obtained at www.ICGtesting.com
Printed in the USA
LVOW01s1745100215

426460LV00003B/598/P